ESSENTIAL NEUROLOGY

Essential

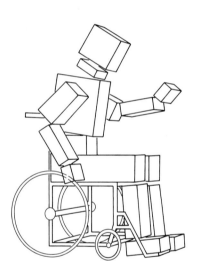

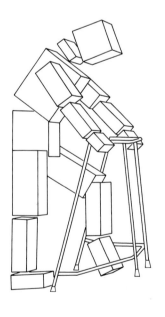

I. M. S. WILKINSON

BSc, MD, MA, FRCP
Consultant Neurologist
Addenbrooke's Hospital
Cambridge
Associate Lecturer
University of Cambridge
Medical School

Neurology

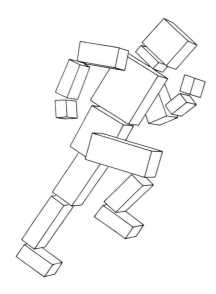

FOUR DRAGONS

OXFORD

BLACKWELL SCIENTIFIC PUBLICATIONS

LONDON   EDINBURGH   BOSTON

MELBOURNE   PARIS   BERLIN   VIENNA

© 1988 and 1989 (Four Dragons) by
Blackwell Scientific Publications
Editorial offices:
Osney Mead, Oxford OX2 0EL
25 John Street, London WC1N 2BL
23 Ainslie Place, Edinburgh EH3 6AJ
3 Cambridge Center, Cambridge,
  Massachusetts 02142, USA
54 University Street, Carlton
  Victoria 3053, Australia

Other Editorial Offices:
Librairie Arnette SA
2, rue Casimir-Delavigne
75006 Paris
France

Blackwell Wissenschafts-Verlag
Meinekestrasse 4
D-1000 Berlin 15
Germany

Blackwell MZV
Feldgasse 13
A-1238 Wien
Austria

First published 1988
Reprinted 1989, 1992
Four Dragons edition 1989
Reprinted 1992

Set by Times Graphics,
Singapore
Printed and bound
in Great Britain
by Redwood Press Ltd
Melksham, Wilts

DISTRIBUTORS

Marston Book Services Ltd
PO Box 87
Oxford OX2 0DT
(*Orders:* Tel: 0865 791155
        Fax: 0865 791927
        Telex: 837515)

USA
Blackwell Scientific
  Publications, Inc.
3 Cambridge Center
Cambridge, MA 02142
(*Orders:* Tel: (800) 759–6102
        (617) 225–0401)

Canada
Times Mirror Professional
  Publishing, Inc.
5240 Finch Avenue East
Scarborough, Ontario M1S 5A2
(*Orders:* Tel: (800) 268–4178
        (416) 298–1588)

Australia
Blackwell Scientific
  Publications (Australia) Pty Ltd
54 University Street
Carlton, Victoria 3053
(*Orders:* Tel: (03) 347 0300)

British Library Cataloguing in
Publication Data

Wilkinson, I.M.S.
  Essential neurology.
  1. Medicine. Neurology
  I. Title
  616.8

  ISBN 0–632–01981–6
  ISBN 0–632–02805–X
  (Four Dragons edition)

To M.K., L.A.L. and M.F.T.Y.
from whom I learnt
a lot about clinical neurology

and to J.B.W.

with whom I'm learning a lot
about everything else

Contents

Preface

Excellent textbooks of neurology already exist, which deal with the subject in a detailed and comprehensive manner. This is not what the majority of clinical medical students require.

In writing this textbook, I have been pre-occupied with the following questions:

- Have I kept to basic principles?
- Have I made each topic as easy as possible to understand, both in the text and in the diagrams?
- Have I omitted all unnecessary detail?

There is no section in the book specifically dedicated to 'How to examine the nervous system'. I believe each student has to learn this by apprenticeship to clinical neurologists in the ward and in the clinic.

Every effort has been made to ensure that this book lives up to its name, in setting out clearly all that the student needs to know about the common neurological and neuro-surgical conditions.

I.W

Chapter 1   Unconsciousness

Introduction and definitions

Patients who become unconscious make their relatives and their doctors anxious. A structured way of approaching the unconscious patient is useful to the doctor so that he behaves rationally and competently when those around him are becoming alarmed.

Unconsciousness is difficult to define. Most people know what is meant by the word. One way of defining unconsciousness is by asking the reader how he would recognize that a person he had just found was unconscious. Answers to this question would probably include statements like this, 'in a deep sleep, eyes closed, not talking, not responding to his name or instructions, not moving his limbs even if you slap him or shake him.'

In terms of neurophysiology and neuroanatomy, it is not completely clear on what consciousness depends. Consciousness involves the normally functioning cerebrum responding to the arrival of visual, auditory, and somatic afferent stimulation as shown in Fig. 1.1.

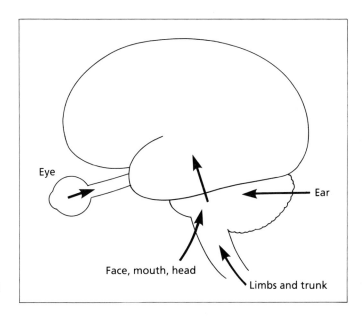

Fig. 1.1. Diagram to show important factors maintaining consciousness.

The ideal circumstances for normal loss of consciousness, in sleep, are entirely compatible with this concept — eyes closed in a darkened room, where it is quiet, in a bed where the body is comfortable, warm and still.

Abnormal states of unconsciousness occur if there is some generalized impairment of cerebral hemisphere function preventing the brain from responding to normal afferent stimulation, or if the cerebral hemispheres are deprived of normal afferent stimulation due to pathological lesions in the midbrain/pons/medulla, blocking incoming visual, auditory and somatic sensory stimuli. The concept of unconsciousness being the consequence of either a diffuse cerebral problem, or a major midbrain/pons/medulla lesion, or both, is useful from the clinical point of view.

A patient may present to the doctor with attacks of unconsciousness between which he feels well, i.e. blackouts, or be in a state of ongoing unconsciousness which persists and demands urgent management, i.e. persistent coma. We will consider these two situations separately.

Fig. 1.2. Diagram to show the common causes of blackouts.

Generalized cerebral malfunction	Severe localized brainstem lesion

Vasovagal syncope Postural hypotension Hyperventilation Cardiac dysrhythmia	Transient ischaemic attacks in the vertebro-basilar circulation
	**Both generalized cerebral and brainstem lesion** 
Hypoxia Hypoglycaemia	Centrencephalic (primary generalized) epilepsy
	Neither generalized cerebral nor brainstem lesion  Psychologically mediated (hysterical) attacks

Attacks of unconsciousness or blackouts

Here it is most likely that the patient, feeling perfectly well, will consult the doctor about some blackouts which have been occurring. Very often a relative will be with him, since the attack has caused as much anxiety in the witnessing relative as in the patient. It is not common for doctors to witness transient blackouts in patients, for obvious reasons. *The value of a competent witness's account is enormous in forming a diagnosis. Arriving at a firm diagnosis in a patient who has suffered unwitnessed attacks is often much more difficult.*

The common causes of blackouts are illustrated in Fig. 1.2.

Causes of blackouts

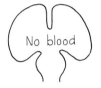

Vasovagal syncope

As a consequence of increased vagal and decreased sympathetic activity, the heart slows and blood pools peripherally. Cardiac output decreases and there is inadequate perfusion of the brain when the patient is in the upright position. He loses consciousness, falls, becomes horizontal, venous return improves, cardiac output improves and consciousness is restored. The attack is worse if the patient is held upright and it is relieved or prevented by lowering the patient's head below the level of the heart.

The distinguishing features of vasovagal syncope are as follows:
• they are more common in teenage and young adult life;
• they may be triggered by standing for a long time, and by emotionally upsetting circumstances (hearing bad news, hearing or seeing explicit medical details, experiencing minor medical procedures, e.g. venipuncture, sutures);
• the patient has a warning of dizziness, visual blurring, feeling hot or cold, sweating, pallor;
• the patient is unconscious for a short period (e.g. 0.5–2 minutes) only, during which time he is flaccid;
• the patient feels nauseated and sweaty on recovery, but is back to normal within 15 minutes or so.

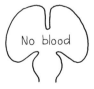

Postural hypotension

In circumstances of decreased sympathetic activity affecting the heart and peripheral circulation, the normal cardio-acceleration and peripheral vasoconstriction that occurs when changing from the supine to the erect position does not occur, and cardiac output and cerebral perfusion are inadequate in the standing position, resulting in loss of consciousness. The situation rectifies itself as described above in vasovagal syncope. The cause of the decreased sympathetic activity is usually pharmacological (overaction of antihypertensive agents or as a side-effect of very many drugs given for other purposes), though it is occasionally due to a physical lesion of the sympathetic pathways in the central or peripheral nervous system.

Clinically, postural hypotension should be suspected as the cause of blackouts if:
- the patient is middle-aged or elderly, and is taking medication of some sort;
- the patient has Parkinson's disease or peripheral neuropathy (the most common physical disorders to be associated with impaired sympathetic innervation);
- the patient complains of dizziness or lightheadedness when standing;
- the attacks occur only in the standing position and can be aborted by sitting or lying down;
- the patient's systolic blood pressure is lower by 30 mmHg or more when in the standing position than when supine.

Hyperventilation

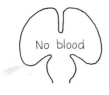

Patients who overbreathe, wash out carbon dioxide from their blood. Arterial hypocapnia is a very strong cerebral vasoconstrictive stimulus. The patient starts to feel light-headed and may lose consciousness. During coma, respiration is quiet and the blood gases return to normal, allowing cerebral blood flow to come back to normal and consciousness to return.

The clues to hyperventilation being the cause of blackouts are:
- the patient is young and female;
- the patient is in a state of anxiety;
- the patient mentions that she has difficulty in 'getting her breath' as the attack develops;
- distal limb paraesthesiae and/or tetany are mentioned (due to the increased nerve excitability which occurs when the concentration of ionized calcium in the plasma is reduced during respiratory alkalosis);
- the attacks can be culminated by rebreathing into a paper bag;
- the symptoms are reproducible by voluntary hyperventilation.

Cardiac dysrhythmia

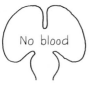

When left ventricular output is inadequate because of either cardiac tachy-arrhythmia or brady-arrhythmia, cardiac output and cerebral perfusion may be inadequate to maintain consciousness. The cardiac arrhythmia is most usually (but not exclusively) caused by ischaemic heart disease. The most classical form of this condition, known as the Adams-Stokes attack, occurs when there is impaired atrio-ventricular conduction leading to periods of very slow ventricular rate and/or asystole.

That cardiac arrhythmia is responsible for the blackouts is suggested by the following features:
- the patient is middle-aged or elderly;
- the attacks are unrelated to posture;
- there is a history of ischaemic heart disease;
- the patient has noticed palpitations;
- episodes of dizziness and presyncope occur as well as episodes in which consciousness is lost;
- marked colour change and/or loss of pulse have been observed by witnesses during the attacks;
- the patient has a rhythm abnormality at the time of examination;
- ischaemic, rhythm or conduction abnormalities are present in the ECG.

Hypoxia

Hypoxia is a very uncommon cause of attacks of unconsciousness. Even in patients with severe respiratory embarrassment, e.g. major asthmatic attack, consciousness is usually retained.

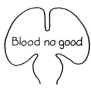

Hypoglycaemia

Except in diabetic patients who are taking oral hypoglycaemic agents or insulin, hypoglycaemia is another very uncommon cause of blackouts. This is because alternative causes of hypoglycaemia (e.g. insulinoma of the pancreas) are rare.

Amongst diabetics, hypoglycaemia should be high on the list of possible causes of blackouts.

Hypoglycaemic attacks:
- may be heralded by feelings of hunger and emptiness;
- are associated with the release of adrenaline (one of the body's homeostatic mechanisms to release glucose from liver glycogen stores in the face of hypoglycaemia). This explains the palpitations, tremor and sweating that characterize hypoglycaemic attacks;
- may not proceed to full loss of consciousness; they may simply cause episodes of abnormal speech, confusion or unusual behaviour;

5   *Unconsciousness*

- may proceed quite rapidly through faintness and drowsiness to coma, especially in children;
- are most conclusively proved by recording a low blood glucose level during an attack, but clearly this is not always possible.

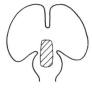

Vertebro-basilar transient ischaemic attacks

Thrombo-embolic material, derived from the heart or proximal large arteries in the chest and neck, may lodge in the small arteries which supply the brainstem. They may cause ischaemia of the brainstem tissue until lysis or fragmentation of the thrombo-embolic material occurs, after which normal perfusion and function of the brainstem returns. It is difficult to know how commonly this mechanism causes blackouts. One reason for this uncertainty is the great difficulty of proving that this is the nature of a patient's attacks.

Vertebro-basilar ischaemia is suggested:
- if the patient is middle-aged or elderly;
- if the patient is known to be arteriopathic (i.e. history of myocardial infarction, angina, intermittent claudication, or stroke);
- if the patient is having transient ischaemic attacks that do not involve loss of consciousness, e.g. episodes of monocular blindness, speech disturbance, hemiplegia, hemianaesthesia, diplopia, ataxia, etc.;
- by the presence of a definite source of emboli, e.g. recent myocardial infarction, atrial fibrillation, neck bruits and asymmetrical values for blood pressure in the patient's arms.

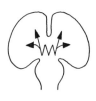

Epilepsy

Chapter 2 deals with epilepsy in detail. Epilepsy may be primary generalized (centrencephalic), in which the abnormal electrical activity starts in deep midline structures (the upper brainstem) and immediately spreads to all parts of both cerebral hemispheres. This is the nature of 'idiopathic' grand mal and petit mal epilepsy, and such a disturbance of brainstem and cerebral hemisphere function is always associated with loss of consciousness.

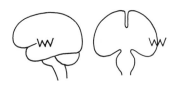

The other main type of epilepsy is focal epilepsy, in which the abnormal electrical activity is localized to one area of the cerebral cortex. In such attacks, there is grossly deranged function in that part of the brain where the epileptic activity is occurring, whilst the rest of the brain remains as normal as possible. No deep midline disturbance occurs, so consciousness is maintained. It is only when focal epileptic activity occurs in the temporal lobe, when local cerebral activity subserving memory is perturbed by the attack, that patients seek help for blackouts which they cannot properly remember. Memory, rather than consciousness, is lost in such attacks.

'Hysterical' attacks

Some patients attract attention to themselves, at a conscious or unconscious level, by having blackouts. The attacks may consist of apparent loss of consciousness and falling, sometimes with simulated convulsive movement of the limbs and face. The patient may claim no memory or awareness during the attack, or he may acknowledge awareness at a very distant level without any ability to respond to his environment or control his body during the attack.

Such psychologically mediated attacks:
• are more common in teenage and young adult life;
• may be suggested by lack of self-injury, and by the coordinated purposeful kind of movements which are witnessed in the attacks;
• may occur in association with genuinely physically caused attacks. It is easy to understand why a young person with epilepsy might respond to adversity by having more 'attacks' rather than by developing some other psychosomatic disorder.

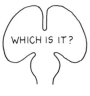

Making the diagnosis in a patient with blackouts

Making the diagnosis is best achieved by giving oneself enough time to talk to the patient so that he can describe all that happens before, during and after the attacks, and similarly by talking to a witness so that he can describe all the observable phenomena of the patient's attack. Physical examination of the patient with blackouts is very frequently normal, so it cannot be relied upon to yield very much information of use. Occasionally, it may be necessary to admit the patient to hospital so that the attacks may be observed by medical and nursing staff.

The investigations that may prove valuable in patients with blackouts are:
• EEG (electroencephalography) and ECG (electrocardiography), with prolonged monitoring of the brain and heart by these techniques, if the standard procedures are not diagnostic;
• blood glucose and blood gas estimations (ideally at the time of the attacks) may help to prove either hypoglycaemia or hyperventilation as the basis of the attacks.

7   *Unconsciousness*

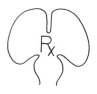

Treatment of the common causes of blackouts

Apart from a general explanation of the nature of the attacks to the patient and his family, there are two other aspects of management.

Specific treatment suggestions

Vasovagal syncope: lower head at onset.

Postural hypotension: remove offending drug, consider physical and pharmacological methods of maintaining the standing blood pressure (tight elastic stockings, fludrocortisone).

Hyperventilation: exercises to control breathing.

Cardiac dysrhythmia: pharmacological or implanted pacemaker control of cardiac rhythm.

Hypoglycaemia: attention to drug regime in diabetics, removal of insulinoma in the rare instances of their occurrence.

Vertebro-basilar TIAs: treat source for emboli, aspirin.

Epilepsy: anticonvulsant drugs.

'Hysterical' attacks: try to establish the reason for this behaviour, and careful explanation to the patient.

Care of personal safety

People who are subject to sudden episodes of loss of consciousness:
- should not *drive motor vehicles;*
- may not be safe in some *working environments* which involve working at heights, using power tools, working amongst heavy unguarded machinery, working with electricity wires;
- may have to curtail some *recreational activities* involving swimming or heights.

A firm but sympathetic manner is necessary in pointing out these aspects of the patient's management.

Before leaving the causes of blackouts, there are two rare neurological conditions to mention briefly. One condition predisposes the patient to frequent short episodes of sleep, *narcolepsy,* and the other gives rise to infrequent episodes of selective loss of memory, *transient global amnesia.* The mechanism of each of these uncommon syndromes is not understood.

Narcolepsy

In this condition, which is familial and very strongly associated with the possession of HLA type DR2, the patient has a tendency to sleep for short periods, e.g. 10–15 minutes. The sleep is just like ordinary sleep to the observer, but is unnatural in its duration and in the strength with which it overtakes the patient. Such episodes of sleep may occur in circumstances where ordinary people feel sleepy, but narcoleptic patients also go to sleep at very inappropriate times, e.g. whilst talking, eating or driving.

The condition is associated with some other unusual phenomena:
• *cataplexy:* transient loss of tone and strength in the legs at times of emotional excitement, particularly laughter and annoyance, leading to falls without any impairment of consciousness;
• *sleep paralysis:* the frightening occurrence of awakening at night unable to move any part of the body for a few moments;
• *hypnogogic hallucinations:* visual hallucinations of faces occurring just before falling asleep in bed at night.

Narcolepsy, and its associated symptoms, are helped by dexamphetamine and the tricyclic agent, clomipramine.

Transient global amnesia

This syndrome, which tends to occur in patients over the age of 50, involves loss of memory for a few hours. During the period of amnesia, the patient cannot remember recent events, and does not retain any new information at all. All other neurological functions are normal. The patient can talk, write, and carry out complicated motor functions (e.g. driving) normally. Throughout the episode, the patient repeatedly asks the same questions of orientation. Afterwards, the person is able to recall all events up to the start of the period of amnesia, remembers nothing of the period itself, and has a somewhat patchy memory of the first few hours following the episode.

Transient global amnesia may occur a few times in a patient's life.

Persistent coma

Assessment of conscious level

The observations that might be made by someone who finds an unconscious body were mentioned at the beginning of

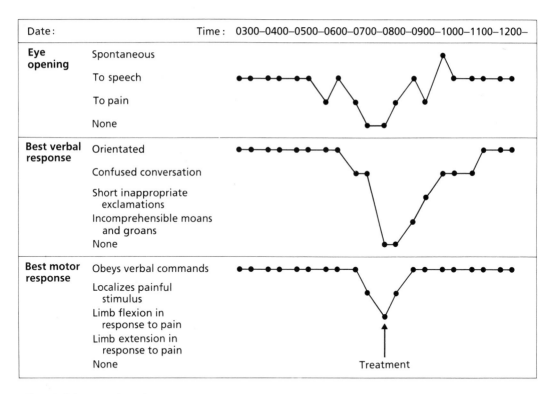

Date:		Time:	0300–0400–0500–0600–0700–0800–0900–1000–1100–1200–
Eye opening	Spontaneous		
	To speech		
	To pain		
	None		
Best verbal response	Orientated		
	Confused conversation		
	Short inappropriate exclamations		
	Incomprehensible moans and groans		
	None		
Best motor response	Obeys verbal commands		
	Localizes painful stimulus		
	Limb flexion in response to pain		
	Limb extension in response to pain		
	None		Treatment

Fig. 1.3. Scheme to show the Glasgow Coma Scale. (After Teasdale G. & Jennett B. (1974) *Lancet* **ii**, 81–3.)

Regulation of pupils

Regulation of Temp.
BP
Pulse
Resp.

Fig. 1.4. Diagram to show important functions of the brainstem.

this chapter: 'in a deep sleep, eyes closed, not talking, not responding to instructions, not moving even when slapped or shaken'. These natural comments have been brought together and elaborated in the Glasgow Coma Scale. This is used very effectively to indicate a patient's level of unconsciousness. It achieves this more objectively than descriptive terms such as 'in a light coma' through to 'profoundly unconscious'. The Glasgow Coma Scale records the level of stimulus required to make the patient open his eyes and also records the patient's best verbal and motor responses, as shown in Fig. 1.3.

The responses of the Glasgow Coma Scale depend upon the cerebrum's response to afferent stimulation. This may be impaired either because of impaired cerebral hemisphere function or because of a major brainstem lesion interfering with access of such stimuli to the cerebral hemispheres. (Lesions in the brainstem that leave access to the cerebrum intact, but block the motor responses from a normally functioning cerebrum, do occur, but are exceedingly rare — the so-called 'locked-in' syndrome.) Direct evidence that there is a major brainstem lesion may be evident in an unconscious patient (Fig. 1.4). Dilatation of the pupils and lack of pupillary constriction to light indicate problems in the midbrain, i.e. 3rd cranial nerve dysfunction. Impaired regulation of body temperature, blood pressure, pulse and

	Mechanism of coma	Cause of coma	Assessment of coma	
	Generalized impairment of cerebral hemisphere function, leading to a sub-standard response to normal afferent stimulation	Overdose of CNS sedative drugs Severe alcoholic intoxication Diabetic comas Renal failure Hepatic failure	Glasgow Coma Scale works really well in these patients, since there is no focal neurological damage, and therefore no lateralizing or focal signs. In severe instances, the noxious process may involve the brainstem as well as the cerebral hemispheres. Signs of depressed brainstem function appear ... impaired pupils and impaired regulation of vital functions	In these patients, the assessment of eyes, speech and motor responses, needed for the Glasgow Coma Scale, is somewhat interfered with, because of the presence of the primary neurological deficit produced by the primary CNS pathology. In such instances, the best eye, speech and limb response which can be achieved (in either of the two eyes, or in any of the four limbs) is the one which is used for the Coma Scale assessment. Despite this interference the Coma Scale, charted at intervals as shown in Fig. 1.3, provides a very valuable guide to an unconscious patient's progress
	Major primary pathology in the brainstem, depriving the cerebral hemispheres of their normal afferent stimulation	Brainstem infarction by basilar artery occlusion Brainstem haemorrhage, as occurs in severe hypertension	These patients have a multitude of abnormal neurological signs, since the major brainstem lesion is causing malfunction in the: • descending motor pathways • ascending sensory pathways • pathways to and from the cerebellum • cranial nerve nuclei • centres regulating vital functions	
	Unilateral cerebral hemisphere mass lesion, causing downward herniation of the medial part of the temporal lobe through the tentorial hiatus, which results in a sideways and downward shift of the brainstem. This situation of secondary brainstem malfunction is one form of 'coning', and is the explanation of coma in such patients. It may become associated with medullary coning at foramen magnum level, as below, if the mass lesion is left untreated	Haematoma Abscess Tumour	These patients have the signs of a unilateral cerebral hemisphere lesion and raised intracranial pressure (papilloedema). In addition the signs of coning (pupillary dilatation and impaired regulation of vital functions) may appear	
	Generalized impairment of cerebral hemisphere function, associated with bilateral cerebral hemisphere swelling. Bilateral medial temporal herniation occurs. Downward shift of the brainstem occurs at the level of the midbrain (tentorial hiatus) and at the level of the medulla (foramen magnum). These patients are in coma because of generalized impairment of cerebral hemisphere function, and because of coning at midbrain and medullary levels	Brain trauma Meningo-encephalitis Cerebral anoxia or ischaemia Status epilepticus	These patients have the signs of bilateral cerebral hemisphere malfunction and raised intracranial pressure (papilloedema). They too may show signs of coning	

Fig. 1.5. Scheme to show the common causes of coma.

respiration may all indicate trouble in the pons/medulla, where the centres controlling these vital functions exist.

When confronted with a patient in coma, a well-trained doctor will assess:
• vital functions of respiration, temperature control, pulse and blood pressure;
• pupil size and reactivity;
• the patient's eyes, speech and motor responses according to the Glasgow Coma Scale.

This approach to the assessment of conscious level holds good regardless of the particular cause of coma in any individual patient.

Causes of coma

In considering the causes of coma it is helpful to think again in terms of disease processes which impair cerebral hemisphere function generally on the one hand, and in terms of lesions in the brainstem blocking afferent stimulation of the cerebrum on the other. The common causes of coma are illustrated in this way in Fig. 1.5.

There is a simple mnemonic to help one to remember the causes of coma (see Fig. 1.6).

	A	E	I	O	U
A = Apoplexy		Brainstem infarction Intracranial haemorrhage			
E = Epilepsy		Post-ictal or inter-ictal coma Status epilepticus			
I = Injury		Concussion — to major head injury			
I = Infection		Meningo-encephalitis Cerebral abscess			
O = Opiates		Standing for all CNS depressant drugs, including alcohol			
U = Uraemia		Standing for all metabolic causes for coma. Quite a useful way of remembering all possibilities here is to think of coma resulting from extreme deviation of normal blood constituents			
		Oxygen		Anoxia	
		Carbon dioxide		Carbon dioxide narcosis	
		Hydrogen ion		Diabetic keto-acidosis	
		Glucose		Hypoglycaemia	
		Urea		Renal failure	
		Ammonia		Liver failure	
		Thyroxine		Hypothyroidism	

Fig. 1.6. A simple mnemonic for the recall of the causes of coma.

Investigation and management of a patient in coma

1 Check that the patient's airway is clear, that breathing is satisfactory, and that the patient's colour is good.

2 Assess the level of coma, looking at vital functions, pupils and items of the Glasgow Coma Scale as mentioned above.

3 Try to establish the cause of the coma by taking a history from relatives or witnesses, physical examination and appropriate tests. It is obviously important to have the common causes of coma (A, E, I, O, U) clearly in one's mind whilst asking the questions, performing the physical examination and ordering investigations.

4 Remember the danger of lumbar puncture in patients in whom coning is imminent or present. Reduction of the CSF pressure below the foramen magnum may encourage further downward herniation at tentorial or foramen magnum level, so *no lumbar puncture if papilloedema is present* is a safe guiding principle.

5 Treat the specific cause of the coma as soon as this is established, e.g. anticonvulsants for epilepsy, antibiotics for meningitis, intravenous glucose for hypoglycaemia.

6 Establish the routine care of an unconscious patient regardless of the cause (see Fig. 1.7).

(a) Observations: assessment every 15–30 minutes of vital functions, pupils, Glasgow Coma Scale, so that improvement or deterioration in the patient's condition can be closely monitored.

(b) Airway, ventilation, blood gases.

(c) Blood pressure, to maintain adequate perfusion of the body, particularly of the brain and kidneys.

(d) Fluid and electrolyte balance.

(e) Nutrition and feeding.

(f) Avoidance of sedative or strong analgesic drugs.

(g) General nursing care of eyes, mouth, bladder, bowels, skin and pressure areas, passive limb mobilization to prevent venous stagnation and contractures, chest physiotherapy.

Fig. 1.7. Diagram to show the routine care of the unconscious patient.

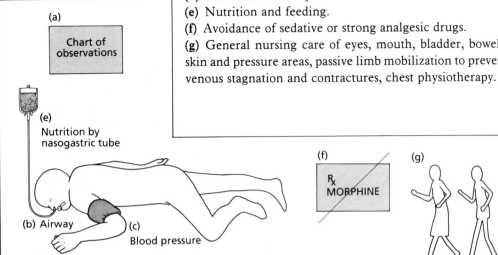

(a) Chart of observations

(e) Nutrition by nasogastric tube

(b) Airway

(c) Blood pressure

(d) Electrolytes

(f) R~x~ MORPHINE

(g) Nurse   Physio

Prognosis for coma

Patients whose coma has been caused by drug overdose may remain deeply unconscious for prolonged periods and yet have a satisfactory outcome. They may need respiratory support during their coma if brainstem function is depressed, but proceed to make a full recovery.

Prolonged coma from other causes has a much less satisfactory outcome. As an example of this, if one takes a group of unconscious patients, whose coma is not due to drug overdose, who
- show no eye opening (spontaneous or to voice),
- express no comprehensible words,
- fail to localize painful stimuli,
- remain like this for more than 6 hours,

more than 50% of them will die, and recovery to independent existence will occur in a minority of the rest. This

Fig. 1.8. Scheme to show the guidelines that exist to help identify those patients who have undergone brainstem death whilst in coma.

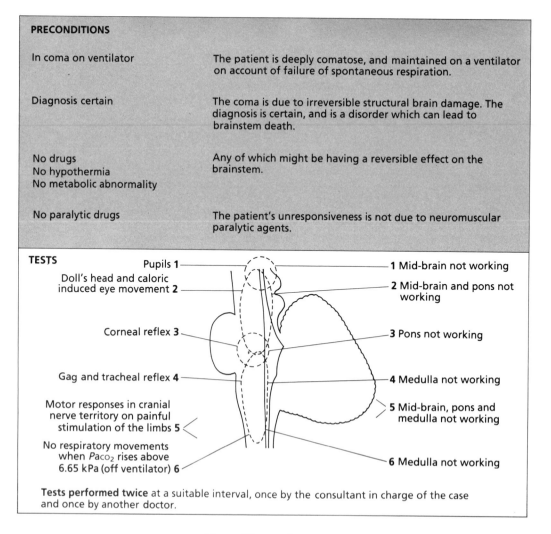

PRECONDITIONS	
In coma on ventilator	The patient is deeply comatose, and maintained on a ventilator on account of failure of spontaneous respiration.
Diagnosis certain	The coma is due to irreversible structural brain damage. The diagnosis is certain, and is a disorder which can lead to brainstem death.
No drugs No hypothermia No metabolic abnormality	Any of which might be having a reversible effect on the brainstem.
No paralytic drugs	The patient's unresponsiveness is not due to neuromuscular paralytic agents.

TESTS

Pupils **1** — 1 Mid-brain not working

Doll's head and caloric induced eye movement **2** — 2 Mid-brain and pons not working

Corneal reflex **3** — 3 Pons not working

Gag and tracheal reflex **4** — 4 Medulla not working

Motor responses in cranial nerve territory on painful stimulation of the limbs **5** — 5 Mid-brain, pons and medulla not working

No respiratory movements when $Paco_2$ rises above 6.65 kPa (off ventilator) **6** — 6 Medulla not working

Tests performed **twice** at a suitable interval, once by the consultant in charge of the case and once by another doctor.

background knowledge must remain in the doctor's mind when counselling relatives of patients in coma, and when planning the care of patients in prolonged coma.

Brainstem death

Deeply unconscious patients whose respiration has to be maintained on a ventilator, whose coma is not caused by drug overdose, clearly have a worsening prognosis as each day goes by. Amongst this group of patients, there will be some who have a zero prognosis, whose brainstems have been damaged to such an extent that they will never breathe spontaneously again.

Guidelines exist to help doctors identify patients who have undergone brainstem death whilst in coma which has been supported by intensive care and mechanical ventilation (Fig. 1.8).

Chapter 2   Epilepsy

Words and definitions

The word epilepsy conjures up something rather frightening and undesirable in most people's minds, because of the apprehension created in all of us when somebody temporarily loses control of his body, especially if unconsciousness, violent movement and impaired communication are involved. Epilepsy is the word used to describe a tendency to episodes, in which a variety of clinical phenomena may occur, which are caused by abnormal electrical discharge in the brain, between which the patient is his normal self. What actually happens to the patient in an epileptic attack depends upon the nature of the electrical discharge, in particular upon its location and duration.

The most major form of epilepsy, which involves sudden unconsciousness and violent movement often followed by coma, is called grand mal. Unless otherwise stated, mention of an epileptic attack would generally infer the occurrence of an episode of grand mal.

Amongst patients and doctors a single epileptic attack may be called an epileptic fit, a fit, an epileptic seizure, an epileptic convulsion or a convulsion. The words tend to be used synonymously. This is a somewhat inaccurate use of words since a convulsion (violent irregular movement) is one component of some forms of epilepsy. There is also a tendency to use the word petit mal for any form of epilepsy which is not too massive or prolonged, even though petit mal really has a rather restricted and specific meaning. Patients and their parents and families very often use softer words other than epilepsy, fits, seizures, or convulsions, which is quite natural. Within families, words like blackout, episode, funny do, attack, blank spell, dizzy turn, fainting spell, trance, daze, petit mal abound when describing epileptic attacks.

We can see that the use of words is often imprecise here. 'A minor fit' may mean one thing to one person and another thing to somebody else, and it may certainly be used by a patient or relative to describe any form of epileptic or nonepileptic attack. We must be tolerant of this amongst patients, but there is always a need to clarify exactly what has happened in an individual attack in an individual patient. Errors in management rapidly appear when the doctor does not know the precise features of each of the patient's attacks.

The last area of semantic difficulty is that the word epilepsy is generally used to indicate a tendency to suffer from epileptic attacks, i.e. more than one attack and perhaps an ongoing tendency. Some medical and non-medical people are upset by the use of the word epilepsy when applied to someone who has only ever had one epileptic attack.

Common forms of epilepsy

Epileptic attacks which are the consequence of electrical discharge starting in the upper midbrain structures and immediately involving all parts of both cerebral hemi spheres are manifestations of *primary generalized or centrencephalic* (middle of the brain) *epilepsy* (see Fig. 2.1).

It is not possible to remain conscious of one's environment during this sort of electrical activity.

There is no demonstrable structural brain abnormality in such cases of epilepsy, and the common kinds of primary generalized or idiopathic epilepsy are *grand mal* and *petit mal.*

If the primary site of abnormal electrical discharge is

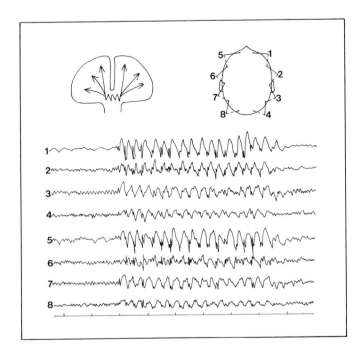

Fig. 2.1. EEG recording typical of centrencephalic or primary generalized epilepsy.

situated in one area of the cortex in one cerebral hemisphere, the patient will be prone to attacks of *focal epilepsy*. The focal nature of the epilepsy may show itself in three ways.

1 *Focal attacks,* where the patient suffers transient episodes entirely due to the abnormal localized epileptic discharge, e.g. focal motor twitching of the right side of the face (see Fig. 2.2).

2 Attacks in which the abnormal electrical discharge starts focally as above, but then spreads over the surface of the cerebral hemisphere and then triggers generalized epileptic discharge involving all parts of both cerebral hemispheres (see Fig. 2.3).

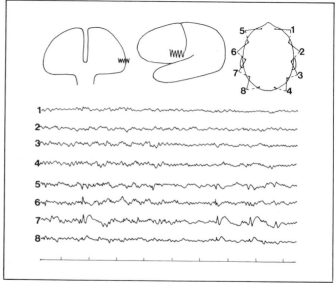

Fig. 2.2. EEG recording typical of focal epilepsy. In this figure, the focal EEG abnormality might generate focal motor twitching of the right side of the face.

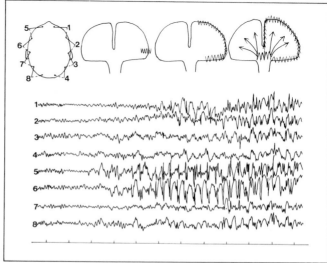

Fig. 2.3. EEG recording which shows epileptic discharge beginning focally, spreading over the surface of the cerebral hemisphere, to trigger generalized epileptic discharge.

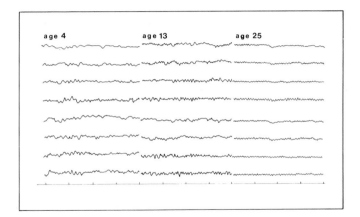

Fig. 2.4. EEG recordings which show the progressive stabilization that occurs with age.

As an example of such an attack, focal convulsive twitching movement, which starts in the right side of the face, spreads to involve the whole of the right side of the body before initiating generalized convulsions throughout the whole body, just as in grand mal. These are known as *Jacksonian attacks* (after Hughlings Jackson who described this gradual spread of focal epileptic activity) or as *grand mal with a stereotyped aura* if the initial focal features last only for a few moments before triggering grand mal.

3 The main indication that a grand mal attack has a focal cause and that the patient does not suffer from primary generalized epilepsy sometimes occurs *after* the fit rather than before it. A grand mal fit which is followed by a focal neurological deficit (e.g. weakness of the right side of the body), lasting for an hour or two, strongly indicates a localized cortical cause for the fit (in or near the left motor cortex in this example). The tell-tale post-epileptic unilateral weakness is known as *Todd's paresis*.

NB Any indication that a patient's epilepsy is focal should lead to a search for an explanation of localized cortical pathology, i.e. Why is this area of cerebral cortex behaving in this way? What is wrong with it?

The young, immature brain of children is less electrically stable than that of adults. This is very clear when comparing the EEG of children and adults (Fig. 2.4). It appears that a child's EEG is made more unstable by fever. Grand mal attacks may occur in children at times of high fever — *febrile convulsions* — and this is certainly another common form of epilepsy.

Grand mal (Fig. 2.5)

- There is no warning.
- *Tonic phase.* The patient suddenly stiffens, as all the muscles in his body enter a state of sustained (tonic)

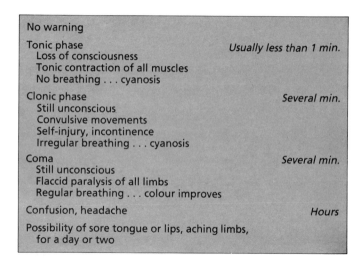

```
No warning

Tonic phase                                    Usually less than 1 min.
    Loss of consciousness
    Tonic contraction of all muscles
    No breathing . . . cyanosis

Clonic phase                                            Several min.
    Still unconscious
    Convulsive movements
    Self-injury, incontinence
    Irregular breathing . . . cyanosis

Coma                                                    Several min.
    Still unconscious
    Flaccid paralysis of all limbs
    Regular breathing . . . colour improves

Confusion, headache                                          Hours

Possibility of sore tongue or lips, aching limbs,
    for a day or two
```

Fig. 2.5. Scheme to show typical severe grand mal epilepsy.

contraction. The limbs are usually straight, the body rather extended, the head and neck extended, the eyes open. The patient falls without any movement of his body to save himself. He loses consciousness as this state of generalized muscular contraction commences. Since the respiratory and laryngeal muscles are involved there is frequently a loud expiratory noise as air is forced out of the chest through tightened vocal cords. There is no breathing during this phase of tonic contraction of all muscles, so cyanosis occurs. The tonic phase does not usually last longer than 30 or 40 seconds, often much less, so that there is just a cry, a fall and stiffening of the whole body before the clonic phase commences.

• *Clonic phase.* Strong, random, disorganized (agonists contracting simultaneously with antagonists) muscular movements occur, involving any and all muscles of the body. These convulsive movements are in no way purposeful, coordinated or predictable. Tongue and lip biting may occur during this phase because the tongue may be protruded at a time when jaw closure occurs, and urinary (even faecal) incontinence frequently happens. Breathing movements occur in the same disorganized way. Synchronization of movement of upper airways, larynx, diaphragm and intercostal muscles is lost. Respiration is jerky, inefficient and noisy. Cyanosis persists. Coordinated swallowing movements do not occur. Saliva (sometimes bloodstained) accumulates in the mouth which, together with the disorganized breathing movements, results in frothing at the mouth. The clonic phase varies in duration from a few seconds to many minutes. It is unusual for this convulsive phase to go on for more than 30 minutes, and it is usually much less.

• *Phase of coma.* After the convulsive movements stop, the patient is in coma. Breathing becomes regular and coordinated. The patient's colour returns to normal so long as the upper airway is clear. The period of time that the patient remains in coma relates to the duration of the previous tonic and clonic phases.

There follows a state of confusion, headache, restlessness and drowsiness before final recovery. This may last for hours. For a day or two, the patient may feel mentally slow and notice aching pains in the limbs subsequent to the convulsive movement.

The description given above is of a severe grand mal attack. They may not be as devastating or prolonged. The tonic and clonic phases may be over in a minute and the patient may regain consciousness within a further minute or two. He may feel like his normal self within an hour or so.

During a grand mal epileptic attack, cerebral metabolic rate and oxygen consumption are increased, yet in the tonic and clonic phases respiration is absent or inefficient with reduced oxygenation of the blood. The brain is unable to metabolize glucose anaerobically, so there is a tendency for accumulation of lactic and pyruvic acid in the brain during prolonged grand mal. This hypoxic insult to the brain with acidosis is the probable cause of post-epileptic (post-ictal) coma.

Petit mal (Fig. 2.6)

As the name implies, a petit mal attack is much less overwhelming and upsetting than a grand mal attack. The attack is sudden in onset, does not usually last longer than 10 seconds, and is sudden in its ending. The patient is usually able to tell that an episode has occurred only because he realizes that a few moments have gone by of which he has been quite unaware. Conversation and events around him have moved on, and he has no recall of the few seconds of missing time.

Observers will note that the patient suddenly stops what he is doing, and that his eyes remain open, distant and staring, possibly with a little rhythmic movement of the eyelids. Otherwise the face and limbs are usually still. The patient remains standing or sitting, but will stand still if the attack occurs while walking. There is no response to calling the patient by name or any other verbal or physical stimulus. The attack ends as suddenly as it commences, sometimes with a word of apology by the patient if the circumstances have been such as to make him realize an attack has occurred.

Whole attack lasts less than 10 seconds

Young person

Sudden onset, sudden end . . . switch-like

Unaware, still, staring

May occur several times a day

Fig. 2.6. Scheme to show typical petit mal epilepsy.

Petit mal usually commences in childhood, so at the time of diagnosis the patient is usually a child or young teenager. It is quite common for petit mal to occur several times a day, sometimes very frequently so that a few attacks may be witnessed during the initial consultation.

Focal epilepsy

The phenomena that occur in focal epileptic attacks entirely depend on the location of the epileptogenic lesion. The most obvious form of focal epileptic attack is when the localized epileptic discharge is in part of the motor cortex (precentral gyrus) of one cerebral hemisphere. During the attack, disorganized strong convulsive movement will occur in the corresponding part of the other side of the body. These are focal motor seizures (see Fig. 2.7).

Figure 2.7 illustrates the common forms of focal epilepsy. *Focal motor seizures, focal sensory seizures* and *adversive seizures* are quite straightforward. *Temporal lobe epilepsy* deserves a special mention, not least because it is probably the commonest form of focal epilepsy. It is necessary to remember what functions reside in the temporal lobe in order to understand what might happen when epileptic derangement occurs in this part of the brain. Apart from speech comprehension in the dominant temporal lobe, the medial parts of both temporal lobes are significantly involved in smell and taste function, and in memory.

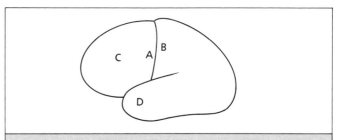

A *Focal motor seizures*
Strong convulsive movements of one part of the contralateral face, body, or limbs

B *Focal sensory seizures*
Strong, unpleasant, slightly painful, warm, tingling, or electrical sensations in one part of the contralateral face, body, or limbs

C *Adversive seizures*
Strong, convulsive turning of the eyes, head, and neck towards the contralateral side (epileptic activity in the frontal eye field)

D *Temporal lobe epilepsy*
Strong, disorganized aberration of temporal lobe function. (see Text and Fig. 2.8)

Fig. 2.7. Scheme to show the common forms of focal epilepsy.

Fig. 2.8. Scheme to show the subjective experiences and objective observations in a patient with temporal lobe epilepsy.

Subjective
  Déjà vu
  Memories rushing through the brain
  Loss of memory during the attack
  Hallucination of smell/taste
  Sensation rising up the body
Objective
  Diminished contact with the environment
  Slow, confused
  Repetitive utterances
  Repetitive movements
  Lip-smacking and sniffing movements

In temporal lobe epileptic attacks, the common subjective experiences are as follows (see also Fig. 2.8):
• memories from the past rush through the head;
• strong and prolonged feelings of *déjà-vu*—the place, the faces, the conversation, etc., have all happened before;
• partial loss of contact with the environment, and inability to remember precise details of what has happened during the attack;
• a strong familiar sense of smell or taste, in the mouth, nose or back of the throat;
• a sensation which is difficult to describe, which is first felt in the abdomen and rises through the chest to end in the throat or head.

In temporal lobe epileptic attacks, it is very common for the subjective experience to be stereotyped, i.e. '... it's always the same, Doctor ...'.

The observer of a patient in a temporal lobe attack may witness the following (see also Fig. 2.8):
• a state of diminished awareness of conversation and environment, the patient appearing confused, somewhat detached from his environment, not properly responsive to the spoken word, physically compliant and rarely aggressive, and unable to carry out any complicated sophisticated activity;
• repetitive, purposeless utterances or limb movements;
• sniffing, smelling, tasting and lip-smacking movements (as the motor concomitants of hallucinations of smell or taste).

Such attacks of rather degraded behaviour and movement are sudden in onset and unprovoked. The patient's overall performance is well below normal in terms of speed and sophistication of thinking and movement. It is not possible for patients to perform activities (criminal or otherwise) requiring quick, complicated thought and action during temporal lobe attacks.

23   *Epilepsy*

Focal epileptic attacks of any kind may remain focal, or the attack may spread and develop into grand mal. When the spread occurs slowly, and especially in the case of focal motor seizures, the attacks are known as *Jacksonian attacks*. When the primary focal disturbance is very transient, especially when it is in the temporal lobe, the momentary focal warning of the grand mal attack tends to be regarded as the *aura*. When focal epilepsy precedes grand mal in this way, there is not usually a tonic phase of grand mal (the focal epilepsy leads straight into the clonic phase). Furthermore the patient himself may or may not be able to remember the focal start of the grand mal attack, especially if this is only transient. The clear focal nature of the attack, e.g. turning of the head and eyes to the right for a few seconds before the grand mal commences, may be apparent only to a witness of the attack. This highlights the cardinal importance of talking to someone who has seen the patient right through an attack.

The focal post-epileptic neurological deficit, *Todd's paresis*, which occasionally indicates the focal nature of the epilepsy, may be apparent to the patient, but is commonly recognized only by a doctor examining the patient shortly after the grand mal attack has ceased.

Febrile convulsions

Grand mal attacks occurring at times of febrile illnesses are not uncommon in children under the age of 5 years. Such attacks are usually transient, lasting a few minutes only. In the majority of cases, the child has only one febrile convulsion, further convulsions in subsequent febrile illnesses being unusual rather than the rule.

A febrile convulsion generates anxiety in the parents. The attack itself is frightening, especially if prolonged, and its occurrence makes the parents wonder if their child is going to have a lifelong problem with epilepsy.

The very small percentage of children with febrile convulsions who are destined to suffer from epileptic attacks unassociated with fever later in life are identifiable to a certain extent by the presence of the following risk factors:
• a family history of non-febrile convulsions in a parent or sibling;
• abnormal neurological signs or delayed development identified before the febrile convulsion;
• a prolonged febrile convulsion, lasting longer than 15 minutes;
• focal features in the febrile convulsion before, during or after the attack.

Rarer forms of epilepsy

Myoclonic jerks

Some patients with primary generalized epilepsy may have attacks of a very sudden jerk movement. This is most commonly seen in younger patients, under the age of 30 years, usually within an hour of waking. The problem affects both arms simultaneously in a single massive sudden movement, causing the patient to drop or throw whatever is in his hands at the time.

Akinetic attacks

Some patients with primary generalized epilepsy suffer from attacks of sudden transient loss of consciousness with loss of muscle power and tone. The patient suddenly blacks out and falls, but within a second or two he is conscious again and struggling to his feet. This is the nature of akinetic attacks. They usually occur in patients who have a severe problem with other sorts of generalized epileptic seizures.

Photosensitive grand mal and petit mal

Some patients with primary generalized epilepsy may be sensitive to rapidly flashing visual stimulation. A large stroboscopic light is the most powerful stimulus but this is not commonly encountered outside the disco hall. Even inside the disco hall the flash frequency is usually too slow for epileptic stimulation. The most common stimuli in modern life to induce this problem are the television set (especially when the patient is very close to the screen) and the large 'space invaders' type of game. Very photosensitive patients may be sensitive to Venetian window blinds and highly coloured striped objects.

Patients with photosensitive epilepsy are usually young, under the age of 30 years, and suffer from grand mal and/or petit mal with or without any visual stimulation. It is only a very small number of patients whose epilepsy occurs only when they are stimulated by flashing or striped stimuli and never happens otherwise.

Hypsarrhythmia or infantile spasms

These are sudden bilateral spasms in which there is flexion of the arms at the shoulders and elbows, occurring in infants often showing developmental delay. The EEG is characteristic and diagnostic.

Status epilepticus

This indicates the occurrence of one epileptic attack after another at very frequent intervals. Petit mal and focal epilepsy may behave in this way, but unless otherwise stated the term status epilepticus indicates the occurrence of one grand mal attack after another without recovery of consciousness between attacks. This is a highly dangerous situation, requiring admission to hospital and probable admission to an intensive care unit.

During grand mal, there exists a state of increased cerebral metabolism and oxygen requirement and decreased respiratory efficiency and cyanosis. Post-epileptic coma is very probably related to this anoxic insult to the brain, with consequent cerebral acidosis. If further grand mal attacks occur at short intervals, it is easy to understand that increasing metabolic acidosis and oedema will occur in the brain, and progressively increasing coma will overtake the patient. Hence, urgent control of seizures and attention to respiration are required in patients with grand mal status.

Table 2.1 Classification of epilepsy

Revised clinical and electro-encephalographic classification of epileptic seizures (*Epilepsia* 1981; **22**:489–501)	Classification of epileptic attacks used in this chapter
Partial seizures	*Focal epilepsy*
(a) simple partial seizure:	Focal attacks, which remain
• motor	localized, in which consciousness
• sensory	is fully preserved, including
• autonomic	temporal lobe epilepsy
(b) complex partial seizure	Focal attacks, which remain localized, in which consciousness is impaired. This mainly applies to the stronger and more intrusive forms of temporal lobe attack
(c) partial seizure evolving to a secondarily generalized tonic–clonic convulsion	Jacksonian attacks Grand mal attacks with a stereotyped aura
Generalized seizures	*Primary generalized epilepsy*
(a) absence seizures	petit mal
(b) myoclonic seizures	myoclonic jerks
(c) clonic seizures	grand mal
(d) tonic seizures	grand mal
(e) tonic–clonic seizures	grand mal
(f) atonic seizures	akinetic attacks
Unclassified epileptic seizures	e.g. hypsarrhythmia

More words and definitions

The classification of epilepsy has always been difficult. There are minor differences in the way epileptic attacks have been arranged in this chapter compared with the most recent international clinical and electro-encephalographic classification of epileptic seizures as shown in Table 2.1.

Diagnosis

Clinical history and the importance of a good witness's account

Certainty of diagnosis in patients with epilepsy depends mainly on the establishment of a clear picture of the features of the attack both from the patient and from a witness. This applies to the diagnosis of any sort of blackout, as emphasized in Chapter 1. One has to go through the precise details of how the patient felt before, during (if conscious) and after the attack, and also obtain a clear description of how the patient behaved during each stage from a witness. One cannot overstate the importance of the clinical history in evaluating attacks. Investigations, such as EEG, should be used to support a diagnostic hypothesis based on the clinical information. Diagnostic certainty is always much more difficult in unwitnessed episodes of loss of consciousness.

The following comments can be made with respect to the differential diagnosis of the different forms of epilepsy.
- *Grand mal* has to be differentiated from the other causes of attacks of loss of consciousness mentioned in Chapter 1. Vasovagal syncope, hyperventilation and psychogenic attacks are more common in younger people, whilst postural hypotension, cardiac dysrhythmia and vertebro-basilar transient ischaemic attacks are more commonly seen in older people. Diabetics on treatment of any sort should prompt one to include hypoglycaemia in the differential diagnosis. In general, tongue and lip biting, irregular noisy breathing, strong convulsive movement, incontinence, post-ictal confusion and limb pains all suggest grand mal.
- *Petit mal* may be confused with absent-minded daydreaming, or with deliberate active inattention of a young person to his environment. The sudden nature of the start and finish of the trance, switch-like, typifies petit mal.
- *Focal motor seizures* do not really have a differential diagnosis.
- *Focal sensory seizures* may be difficult to differentiate from episodes of transient cerebral ischaemia.
- *Adversive seizures* can be confused with oculo-gyric crises,

which are occasionally seen in patients receiving any form of phenothiazine therapy (and a few other drugs). In the latter, the eyes are strongly deviated upwards within the orbits for long periods, whereas both the head and the eyes turn jerkily in adversive seizures, which not infrequently lead to grand mal.

• *Temporal lobe attacks* are strongly suggested by *déjà-vu* and smell or taste phenomena, and diminish in likelihood if the attacks of behavioural disturbance are in any way provoked. Unusual behaviour requiring alert, quick, clear thinking and/or well-coordinated physical movement is more likely to be of psychological than epileptic significance.

Establishing the cause of epilepsy

Apart from accurate information regarding the attacks, there is further information to be elucidated at the interview and examination. If the attacks are thought to be epileptic, an enquiry should be mounted as to the cause of the epilepsy. Primary generalized or idiopathic epilepsy (petit mal, grand mal, myoclonic jerks, photosensitive epilepsy) is familial, so questioning may reveal other members of the family who suffer from epileptic attacks. Any form of focal epilepsy (and some cases of grand mal with no apparent focal features) reflects the presence of intracranial pathology. Most commonly, this pathology is an area of scarring subsequent to some previous active pathology, though sometimes epileptic attacks may occur when the pathological process is in the active phase:

• following birth trauma to the brain;
• following trauma to the skull and brain later in life;
• during or following meningitis, encephalitis or cerebral abscess;
• at the time of, or as a sequel to, cerebral infarction, cerebral haemorrhage or subarachnoid haemorrhage;
• as a result of the inevitable trauma of neurosurgery.

Sometimes, the epileptic attacks are caused by biochemical insults to the brain, rather than by localized physical diseases, such as:

• during alcohol or drug withdrawal;
• during hepatic, uraemic, hypoglycaemic comas;
• whilst on major tranquillizing or antidepressent drugs.

At the front of one's mind must be the possibility that the patient's epilepsy is an early symptom of a brain tumour. Brain tumours are not a common cause of epilepsy, but they are not to be missed. Epilepsy of adult onset, especially if focal and/or associated with evolving abnormal neurological signs, should initiate strong thoughts about the possibility of a tumour.

Physical examination

Physical examination is clearly important since it may reveal abnormal neurological signs which indicate evidence of:
- previous intracranial pathology;
- current intracranial pathology;
- evolving intracranial pathology as indicated above.

EEG and other investigations

The EEG is the most helpful investigation in confirming the diagnosis of epilepsy and in giving commentary as to the focal or generalized nature of the epilepsy (see Figs 2.1–2.3). A routine EEG lasts about 20 minutes and some patients with epilepsy may show no EEG abnormality during this sampling period. Hyperventilation and photic stimulation are known to trigger epileptic activity, and are used routinely to increase the yield of positive information at the time of routine EEG recording in patients with epilepsy. Despite this, approximately 30% of patients with epilepsy may show no abnormality. In these patients, it may be useful either to carry out an EEG during drug-induced sleep (known to make focal epileptic spike activity more prominent), or to perform some form of prolonged recording over hours or even days (which is feasible by recording the EEG onto portable tape-recording equipment worn by the ambulant patient, followed by display and analysis of the recorded information).

Imaging of the brain (e.g. by CT scan) is being carried out increasingly more often in patients with epilepsy. It is unnecessary in patients with primary generalized seizures, idiopathic epilepsy, confirmed by EEG. It is important in other cases of epilepsy, looking for focal intracranial pathology. Imaging is mandatory in the population identified earlier in whom there is a definite possibility of a brain tumour.

In summary therefore, the stages in diagnosis in a patient with epilepsy are:
1 talk to the patient, and to witnesses, about the attacks;
2 wonder why the patient has epilepsy, and what is causing it;
3 examine the patient;
4 investigate the patient, certainly by EEG, and possibly by other techniques.

Management

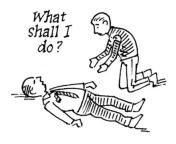

What shall I do?

'On the spot'

If somebody suddenly has a grand mal fit, people close at hand should:

1 look after the patient's airway (by putting the patient into the semisupine position and applying strong upward pressure to the floor of the mouth and chin);

2 prevent self-injury during strong convulsive movements (by keeping the patient away from hard, sharp or hot objects).

Relatives of newly diagnosed epileptic patients certainly appreciate advice of this sort. In an adult, one would generally wait for the convulsions to cease and for the patient to regain consciousness. If one can establish that the patient is subject to epileptic fits, no further medical action is required. If the patient has never had a fit before, and especially if there are focal features to the fits or post-ictal stage, further medical advice will be required either immediately or in the next few days. In children with febrile convulsions, diazepam may be administered *per rectum* if it is available, and further medical attention should be sought if the convulsion has not stopped (with or without diazepam) within five minutes.

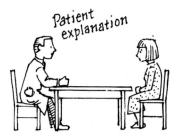

Patient explanation

Explanation

Generally supportive comments and explanation about epilepsy, appropriate to the level of intelligence of the patient and his relatives, constitute the first steps in the management of newly diagnosed epilepsy. The actual word epilepsy greatly upsets some families. It is a good idea to ask the patient and relatives what epilepsy means to them as a starting point for explanation and reassurance. Not uncommonly, it is the relatives, rather than the patient, who are more anxious about attacks involving unconsciousness. They need to be reassured that however serious the appearance of an epileptic attack, patients do not die during them (so long as their airway remains free). Associations of epilepsy with mental subnormality, madness, brain tumours, epileptic 'homes', incurability, transmission to the next generation, etc. are all likely to be introduced during this phase of explanation, and it is important that the doctor has a chance of correcting preconceived ideas in the patient or his family at the outset.

The facts that young people tend to grow out of their tendency to epilepsy, and that epilepsy can be controlled by drugs in the majority of cases, need to be clearly stated.

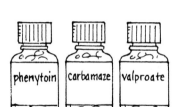

(serum level of anticonvulsants)

Drug therapy

Positive motivation towards taking anticonvulsant drugs, which have side-effects, and which may need to be taken regularly for several years, is not automatic in patients with epilepsy. It will be optimized by careful explanation about the drugs, and allowing time for the patient to express his feelings about the prospect of taking the pills regularly.

Biochemical estimation of serum levels of most of the commonly used anticonvulsants is now available. Their mechanism of action is poorly understood—blood levels do not necessarily indicate brain levels—and the drugs' anticonvulsant properties are unlikely to be a simple function of serum levels. Thus, serum levels must be viewed somewhat circumspectly. If a small dose of an anticonvulsant is controlling an individual's problem with epilepsy, there is no need to use a bigger dose just because the serum level is known to be low. Serum levels are useful, however, in checking compliance, in arriving at an individualized dose in many patients, in keeping anticonvulsant dose in step with bodyweight in growing children, and in avoiding anticonvulsant intoxication.

It was thought that particular forms of epilepsy responded best to particular anticonvulsants. In recent years, this idea of specificity has been substantially disproved. Primary generalized seizures are generally more responsive to drug therapy than any form of focal epilepsy. The commonly used anticonvulsants are listed below:

- as first-line drugs:
  phenytoin;
  carbamazepine;
  sodium valproate;

- as second-line drugs:
  phenobarbitone;
  primidone;
  clonazepam;
  ethosuximide;
  clobazam;
  diazepam.

The pharmacological metabolism and half-life vary from one drug to another. With the exception of phenytoin and phenobarbitone, which are metabolized very slowly and can be given on a once daily schedule, the other anticonvulsants should be given on a twice or thrice daily schedule to achieve satisfactory serum levels throughout the 24 hours. Discussion of timing and establishment of a routine to help compliance are worthwhile activities with individual patients.

The most common toxic effects of the anticonvulsants are drowsiness and a cerebellar syndrome (slurred speech, nystagmus, limb and gait ataxia), but these are usually avoided if the drugs are introduced in modest dosage and gradually increased with serum level control. Most patients do not experience these unwanted effects. Individual anticonvulsants do have specific side-effects (gum hypertrophy, acne, hirsutism with phenytoin; liver cell damage and hair loss with valproate), but these are rarely a major problem in clinical practice. All the anticonvulsants are very weakly teratogenic; this aspect will be discussed later in this chapter.

The use of anticonvulsants does complicate the simultaneous use of two other commonly used drugs: the oral contraceptives and the oral anticoagulant agent, warfarin. This is partly as a result of shared protein-binding sites in the plasma and partly as a result of liver enzyme induction. When anticonvulsants are being used simultaneously with one of these other drugs, larger doses of each are required to achieve the same serum levels and therapeutic effect.

Once anticonvulsant therapy is commenced, it is usual to maintain the treatment for a minimum of 2–3 years. If the attacks are well controlled, after the patient has been fit-free for 2 or 3 years, the drug can be gradually withdrawn over 6–12 months. Often an EEG is performed before withdrawal, confidence about withdrawal being greater if there is no epileptic activity to be found in the EEG.

If control is not established by an anticonvulsant drug and compliance has been established by serum level testing, an alternative anticonvulsant should be used instead of the first. Whenever possible, one drug should be used at a time rather than using several anticonvulsants simultaneously. This is because there is no strong evidence to suggest that two drugs work together better than one, individual anticonvulsant drug metabolisms cross-react with each other, and side-effects are commoner when two or three drugs are used simultaneously.

Sensible restrictions

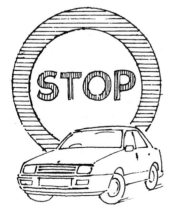

Until satisfactory control of epileptic attacks has been established, and for a little while longer, it is important for patients with most forms of epilepsy to be aware of the dangers of driving, riding a bicycle, heights, open heavy machinery, swimming and water sports. Advice to each patient has to be individualized, bearing in mind the type and frequency of his epileptic attacks. In the UK, the driving licensing authorities have definite guidelines for patients and doctors to follow, and it is the doctor's role to make sure that the patient understands where he stands in relation to these. A patient who has had more than one attack of epilepsy has to refrain from driving until two fit-free years have elapsed, regardless of whether the patient is on medication or not. This is the general rule in the UK, which has exceptions for single attacks, nocturnal attacks and 'provoked' attacks. Very gentle but firm explanation is often required when pointing out the need for these restrictions.

Most patients with photosensitive epilepsy can attend discos where lights flash at rates too slow to stimulate epilepsy. Such patients should avoid video games and sit well back from the TV screen.

Occupation

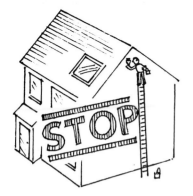

The financial benefits and personal prestige of working are important in the life of a patient with epilepsy, just as for everybody else. Nevertheless, it is more difficult for epileptic people to become employed. Some occupations are completely closed to patients with epilepsy, e.g. jobs requiring an HGV or PSV driving licence and jobs in the armed forces, police or fire services. Some occupations may be very difficult for patients with incompletely controlled epilepsy, e.g. teaching, working with young children, nursing and working near fire or water, at heights, or around unguarded machinery. Individual employers running shops, restaurants, etc. may be unable to accept epileptic attacks amongst their staff.

Special considerations in females with epilepsy

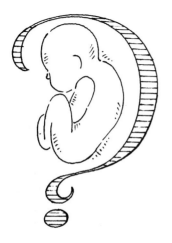

1 As already mentioned, the metabolism and transport systems of anticonvulsant drugs interact with those of oral contraceptive drugs, so special advice and monitoring are necessary if the two sorts of medication are to be taken concurrently.
2 All anticonvulsant drugs are weakly teratogenic, but the risks of stopping all medication and allowing uncontrolled epileptic attacks to occur in early pregnancy are greater to mother and fetus. Furthermore, the metabolism of most anticonvulsant drugs is increased during pregnancy, so drug level monitoring may show the need for slightly increased anticonvulsant dosage during pregnancy.
3 Most anticonvulsants appear in the mother's milk during lactation, but not in quantities that affect the neonate. Mothers on anticonvulsants should be allowed to breast-feed if this is their wish.

4 Focal epilepsy, due to an epileptogenic cortical scar, is not an hereditary condition. Idiopathic, primary generalized, epilepsy is a familial condition so a little genetic counselling may be necessary in such cases. The risk of epilepsy in a child born to a couple, one of whom suffers from idiopathic epilepsy, is small. If both parents suffer from epilepsy, the risk becomes much greater (up to 1 in 4).

5 Care of infants and toddlers may be difficult for a parent who is unlucky enough to suffer from epileptic attacks which remain frequent despite drug therapy.

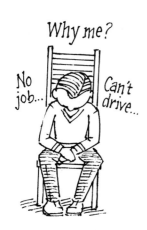

Psychological factors

1 Unpredictable attacks of one sort of or another, the word 'epilepsy', the need to take tablets, restrictions on driving and some recreational activities, exclusion from some occupations and difficulty in obtaining employment may all make patients with epilepsy feel second class, depressed, victimized or aggressive. The size of this psychological reaction is a measure of the patient's personality on the one hand, and of the support and encouragement he receives from his family and doctor on the other.

2 Stress is probably not a major factor in causing individual attacks in a person prone to epileptic fits. It is perfectly natural for patients to look round for causes explaining the occurrence of attacks, but the main difficulty of most patients' epilepsy is its complete unpredictability.

3 Emotional thought and behaviour are aspects of normal temporal lobe function. In patients with abnormal temporal lobes, for whatever reason, there may be some abnormalities of such functions in addition to temporal lobe epilepsy. This is not an inevitable association but it is one to bear in mind when managing patients with this form of epilepsy.

4 If an epileptic patient has difficulty coping with life and develops psychosomatic symptoms, it is quite possible that he will start to have blackouts that are not epileptic but emotional in origin. This may create a diagnostic situation which can be resolved only by admission to hospital for observation and EEG monitoring. It emphasizes the need to establish the precise features of a patient's attacks for correct management.

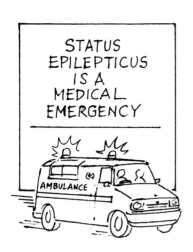

Status epilepticus

Any form of status epilepticus is an indication for hospitalization to establish control of the seizures, but in the case of grand mal status the problem is a medical emergency requiring admission to an intensive care unit. There are three main directions of treatment of grand mal status:

1 routine care of the unconscious patient (see Chapter 1);

2 control of seizure activity in the brain. This means the maintenance of the patient's normal anticonvulsant regime, and the use of additional anticonvulsants given by naso-gastric tube. Very frequently, it is necessary to use intra-venously administered anticonvulsants whose rate of administration can be adjusted to the frequency of fits. The main agents to be used in this way are chlormethiazole, diazepam and occasionally anaesthetic barbiturates, such as thiopentone;

3 maintenance of optimal oxygenation of the blood. This may mean the use of oxygen and an airway, but is quite likely to necessitate paralysis and ventilation. It is important to remember the control of seizure activity in the brain of the paralyzed. Anticonvulsant therapy must be continued. The most sophisticated way to control seizure activity under these circumstances is by the use of some form of EEG monitoring equipment.

Surgical treatment

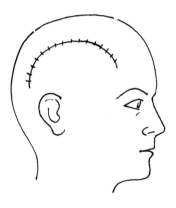

Very occasionally, in a patient with a highly localized epileptogenic focus, which is producing intractable epilep-tic attacks uninfluenced by anticonvulsant drug therapy, the focal area of the brain may be removed with benefit. Surgery of this sort is not performed very frequently. It is more common with foci in the temporal lobes than anywhere else. Meticulous pre-operative and operative EEG recording are required.

Chapter 3   Headache and facial pain

Introduction

Any pain in the head or face must be due to interference with some pain-sensitive structure, and attempts have been made to classify the common forms of headache and face pains in this way. The idea is attractive as a scientific way of approaching the subject, but has little else to commend it. Such an approach does not readily simplify the student's task of familiarizing himself with the common forms of headache and facial pain. It is easier to consider each clinical category of pain in the head or face, and to mention what is known of the relevant pathophysiology in passing.

Tension headache

Tension headache is very common and hard to relieve. It is frequently described as a tight band round the head. It is often constant, without marked diurnal variation. It is usually severe, described in superlatives, and not infrequently the patient pressurizes the doctor to do something to relieve the headache.

    The source of the state of tension, such as in an anxious striving young executive who has become grossly over-committed, or in an inadequate, non-robust person who has difficulty in coping with normal stresses, or in a fairly normal person faced with excessively severe problems, is sometimes apparent at interview but not always.

    Treatment consists of trying to help the patient to understand the nature of his headache, with reassurance that there is no serious physical cause. Modification of life circumstances may be advisable but cannot always be achieved. Analgesic medication is not very helpful. Relaxation therapy (physical and pharmacological) may prove beneficial. It is often difficult to satisfy patients complaining of tension headaches.

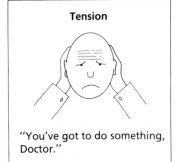

Tension

"You've got to do something, Doctor."

Migraine

Migraine headaches are common in that a significant percentage of the population suffer from them. Patients with migraine are symptom-free most of the time, but suffer episodes of headache from time to time. This is an important characteristic of migraine from the diagnostic point of view.

Migraine is more common in females than males and has usually shown itself by the age of 35 years. It is familial. The interval between attacks is extremely variable, it can be days, weeks, months or years. A few attacks a year would be typical of most patients' migraine.

Some patients notice definite precipitating factors, e.g. food, alcohol, menstrual periods, the contraceptive pill, stress or relief from stress (weekend migraine attacks). The vast majority of sufferers are unable to identify any causative factors.

During an attack, there is a phase of vasoconstriction and reduced blood flow in the cranial arteries, during which time there may be ischaemia of the retinal or cerebral tissue. Flashing lights, coloured lights, and spectra arranged in stereotyped patterns may be seen, though blurring or loss of vision is perhaps more typical. Less commonly, speech disturbance, hemisensory or hemiparetic symptoms may occur during this ischaemic phase. Such neuro-ophthalmological deficits alarm patients when they occur. After the phase of vasoconstriction, which sometimes does not produce sufficient ischaemia to result in symptoms, cerebral vasodilatation and increased cerebral blood flow occur. At this point, the visual or neurological symptoms settle to be replaced by a throbbing headache. This is usually felt at the front of the head, commonly unilaterally or asymmetrically. The headache is often associated with photophobia, nausea, vomiting and general incapacitation so that a patient in a severe attack will want to be alone, in bed, in a darkened room.

The phase of vasoconstriction lasts for less than an hour, often much less; the phase of vasodilatation lasts for hours, occasionally less in children, and sometimes for a day or two in severely affected adults. Some patients know that if they can get to sleep the attack of migraine will come to an end.

What starts the cycle of vasoconstriction followed by vasodilatation in the cranial arteries in patients with migraine remains uncertain. The release of vaso-active amines (e.g. serotonin, noradrenaline) into the blood (perhaps from platelets) may play a part, but why this should occur is not understood.

Patients with migraine have no abnormal physical signs

on examination. Extremely rarely, migraine may be symptomatic of some intracranial vascular anomaly, an arteriovenous malformation. One should consider this rare circumstance if the migraine pain is always on the same side of the head, if some of the features of the attack seem too severe for migraine and bring associated focal epileptic phenomena to mind, and if a cranial bruit can be heard when the stethoscope is applied to the orbit.

The treatment of migraine is mainly pharmacological if a clear precipitant cannot be identified. For an attack of migraine, the patient may respond best to simple/moderate strength analgesics taken with an anti-emetic agent, e.g. aspirin plus metoclopramide. The vasoconstrictive action of ergotamine is often of benefit if it is taken at the very onset of the migraine attack. If vomiting is a pronounced feature of the patient's attacks, the ergotamine may have to be given sublingually, by inhalation or as a suppository. If the neuro-ophthalmological symptoms are very conspicuous, indicating a pronounced ischaemic effect during the vaso-constrictive phase of the attack, ergotamine is best avoided.

Migraine attacks may be made less frequent and less severe by the regular prophylactic administration of clonidine, antiserotonin agents like pizotifen or methysergide, or beta-adrenergic blockers such as propranolol.

Migrainous neuralgia

Migrainous neuralgia is also known as 'cluster headache' because of its usual tendency to occur repetitively over a few weeks, once or twice a day, with long intervals of a year or more until it recurs in the same way. During the few weeks of activity in the condition, episodes of pain last about 30–45 minutes, often at night and often at the same time.

Unlike ordinary migraine, migrainous neuralgia is very much more common in men than women. The pain is very severe, located in the orbit and associated with local redness and swelling, unilateral nasal congestion and lacrimation. The intense pain causes misery whilst it is present and it is difficult to relieve. Its mechanism is not properly understood, but relates to migraine to some extent in that ergotamine-containing compounds are of some help in its relief.

As the time of the pain is predictable to a certain extent, some relief may be achieved by giving the patient a dose of analgesic (such as codeine phosphate) with some ergotamine preparation an hour or so before the anticipated time of the attack. Patients are helped by being reminded that the pains usually settle down spontaneously after a few weeks.

Migrainous neuralgia

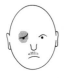

"Mainly at night, I could set the clock by it. Really severe."

Subarachnoid haemorrhage and meningitis

When the meninges are irritated and inflamed, pain is felt throughout the head and neck, especially in the occipital region. Forward flexion of the neck moves the inflamed meninges, and is strongly resisted by the patient. This gives rise to the classical sign of meningeal irritation (meningism) known as 'neck stiffness'.

The headache and neck stiffness are severe and sudden in onset when the meningeal irritation is due to blood in the subarachnoid space (subarachnoid haemorrhage). The symptoms and signs evolve a little more gradually in the case of meningitis caused by pyogenic bacteria and acute viral infection. Evidence of raised intracranial pressure (depression of conscious level, papilloedema) and abnormal neurological signs are not uncommon in patients with subarachnoid haemorrhage and meningitis. Urgent admission to hospital, without the use of strong analgesic drugs (which may further impair the conscious level), for CT head scanning, lumbar puncture, antibiotics, etc., constitute the ideal early management of patients with headache associated with neck stiffness.

Raised intracranial pressure

The precise mechanism of the headache that occurs when intracranial pressure is too high is poorly understood in terms of pain-sensitive structures. The fact that the headache is worst when the patient is lying down makes sense, and is one of the diagnostic characteristics.

The headache of raised intracranial pressure is often present on waking therefore, and sometimes wakes patients from their sleep. The pain is felt all over the head, or towards the back of the head, and may not be too severe. There may be other features of raised intracranial pressure (impairment of conscious level, vomiting, papilloedema), and there may be focal neurological signs due to the causative intracranial space-occupying lesion (haematoma, abscess, neoplasm).

Urgent admission to hospital for investigation *excluding lumbar puncture* is the correct early management of headaches strongly suggestive of raised intracranial pressure.

It is interesting to remember that headache is quite a common symptom of systemic arterial hypertension. How much this type of headache is caused by an elevation of intracranial pressure is a little uncertain. Normally, the cerebral circulation autoregulates to changes in arterial pressure but this autoregulation may fail with sustained high levels of arterial blood pressure, so that intracranial pressure may rise and cause headache. Cerebral vasodilatation caused by arterial hypercapnia may cause headaches which have features of raised intracranial pressure.

After diagnostic lumbar puncture in general clinical practice (not in patients with suspected raised intracranial pressure!), CSF may leak through the hole made in the theca in the lumbar region for several days afterwards. Intracranial pressure is low in these circumstances. The main characteristic of post-lumbar puncture headache is that it is relieved by lying flat and aggravated by the upright position.

Trigeminal neuralgia

Trigeminal neuralgia describes the occurrence of sudden severe transient pains, lasting a moment or two, in the territory of one trigeminal nerve. The pain is unilateral, usually in the maxillary or mandibular territory, close to the mouth or nose. Each stab of pain is severe, like an electric shock, and sudden enough to make the patient jump (hence the french name '*tic douloureux*'). The pain may recur many times a day and tends to be triggered by contact with the skin of the affected area. Cold wind upon the area, washing, shaving, teeth-cleaning, talking, chewing, eating, drinking may all trigger the pain, and the patient may reduce or stop these activities.

Trigeminal neuralgia usually occurs in patients over the age of 55 years, and is unassociated with any abnormal signs. Its occurrence in younger patients and the presence of abnormal signs should make one suspect that the pain is symptomatic rather than idiopathic. Multiple sclerosis (with demyelination in the brainstem), or some compressive lesion of the trigeminal nerve (such as a neuroma or meningioma), are the most likely underlying pathology in the rare instances of symptomatic trigeminal neuralgia.

Ordinary, idiopathic trigeminal neuralgia tends to cause paroxysmal pain for a few months, and then improves spontaneously for a while. In the vast majority of cases, it is helped by carbamazepine. Sometimes, phenytoin is used if control cannot be achieved by tolerable doses of carbamazepine. The response of trigeminal neuralgia to two commonly used anticonvulsants suggests that the condition involves some paroxysmal electrical discharge in the brainstem.

Trigeminal neuralgia that cannot be controlled by drugs may be treated by making lesions (e.g. with injected alcohol) in the branches of the nerve supplying the affected part of

Trigeminal neuralgia

"Sudden cruel severe stabs of pain which make me jump."

the face. Such procedures frequently give significant relief but at a price, since it is very difficult to make a lesion that selectively relieves pain yet leaves sensation intact in the affected area.

Post-herpetic neuralgia

In the face and head, Herpes zoster infection most commonly involves the ophthalmic division of the trigeminal nerve. The condition is painful during the acute vesicular phase, and, in a small percentage of patients, the pain persists after the rash has healed. The occurrence of persistent pain, post-herpetic neuralgia, does not relate to the age of the patient at the time of the infection, nor to the severity of the acute infection. The use of antiviral agents at the time of the acute infection has not been shown to alter the incidence of post-herpetic neuralgia.

Post-herpetic neuralgia can produce a tragic clinical picture. The patient is often elderly (since shingles is more common in the elderly), with evidence of previous infection (thin depigmented areas of skin where the vesicles were at the time of the acute infection), and he is in constant pain. Contact with the affected area of skin aggravates the pain. Not infrequently, the patient becomes very depressed, loses weight and cannot sleep properly.

The pain does not tend to settle. Patients with this condition need a lot of support and encouragement, since the neuralgic pain does not respond to analgesic drugs at all readily. Transcutaneous nerve stimulation (in which a portable battery-operated kit delivers a very light electrical tingling stimulus repetitively to the affected area) is some times helpful in post-herpetic neuralgia, but rarely when it is affecting the face. Nerve section and ablation are occasionally tried, but with mixed results.

Giant cell arteritis

In elderly people, the extracranial and the intra-orbital arteries may become affected by an inflammatory arteritis (in which multinucleate giant cells are to be found), which is painful and dangerous. The danger lies in the fact that the lumen of these arteries may become obliterated because of the thickening of the artery walls and associated thrombosis.

Patients with giant cell arteritis generally feel unwell, short of energy, and apathetic. The condition overlaps with polymyalgia rheumatica, in which similar symptoms are associated with marked stiffness of the muscles (especially around the shoulders, and especially in the mornings).

Post-herpetic neuralgia

"It's been there every day since I had the shingles."

Giant cell arteritis

"I don't feel at all well, Doctor. I can't put my head on the pillow."

The arteritis causes headache and tenderness of the scalp (when resting the head on the pillow, when wearing a hat, and when brushing the hair), because of the inflamed arteries. The superficial temporal arteries may be tender, red, swollen and non-pulsatile. The condition is sometimes known as temporal arteritis because of the very frequent involvement of the superficial temporal arteries, but the facial arteries are often involved (to be felt over the mandible just anterior to the masseter muscles), as are other arteries in the scalp.

The arterial occlusive aspects of the disease chiefly concern the small branches of the ophthalmic artery in the orbit. Sudden and irreversible blindness due to infarction of the distal part of the optic nerve is the main danger. Pain in the jaws when eating may indicate occlusive disease in the facial artery, and occasionally strokes may indicate occlusive disease in the carotid and vertebral arteries in the neck.

Giant cell arteritis is an emergency requiring urgent admission to hospital, for estimation of the ESR (usually above 60 mm/hour), temporal artery biopsy and high-dose steroid treatment. Most patients will continue to need steroids in much diminished doses for a couple of years, and sometimes for much longer.

The main responsibility of the doctor to patients with giant cell arteritis is to think of the condition in elderly people complaining of general ill-health and headache, so that treatment is commenced before irreversible neuro-ophthalmological complications occur.

Subdural haematoma

Elderly people who bang their heads may subsequently develop a collection of blood in the subdural space over the surface of one or other cerebral hemisphere (occasionally over both sides). Symptoms of raised intracranial pressure evolve, often weeks or months after the trauma. The head injury may be so mild as to have been forgotten by the time of presentation. Patients on long-term anticoagulants, and chronic alcoholics who fall from time to time, are two groups of patients predisposed to chronic subdural haematoma.

Slowing of intellectual processes, memory impairment, sleepiness, headaches, physical slowness and unsteadiness are the common features of chronic subdural haematoma. Because the collection of blood is outside the brain, focal neurological signs appear late.

Urgent admission to a neurosurgical unit for CT scanning

Subdural haematoma

"He's sleepy, slow and unsteady. He wet the bed last night."

and for removal of the fluid blood through burrholes constitutes the ideal management of patients with chronic subdural haematoma. Recovery is usually impressive.

Post-concussion syndrome

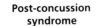

Post-concussion syndrome

" I've not been myself, ever since that accident."

Patients of any age who have an injury to their head resulting in concussion, may suffer a group of symptoms during the months afterwards, even though physical examination and investigation are entirely normal.

The head injury is usually definite but slight, e.g. transient concussion, overnight observations in hospital, no abnormal neurological signs during those observations, and no skull fracture. Subsequently, the patient may complain of headaches (which are frequent or constant), impaired concentration, poor memory, difficulty in taking decisions, irritability, depression, reduced libido, difficulty in sleeping, dizziness and reduced capacity for physical activity. These symptoms, or some of them, may persist for months or even a year or two.

How much these symptoms are physical in origin, how much they are psychological, and precisely how much they relate to medico-legal activity and compensation following the injury is not completely certain, and probably varies a good deal from one patient to another.

Atypical facial pain

Atypical facial pain

"I'm beginning to think I'm neurotic."

Some patients may occasionally present with persistent pains on one side of the face which cause a great deal of misery. The pain does not have the characteristics of migrainous neuralgia or trigeminal neuralgia, the patient is usually younger and female, and physical examination and investigation are completely normal. Like tension headaches, atypical facial pain probably has a psychological basis, and is extremely difficult to relieve. Tricyclic antidepressants are recommended but are often resisted by the patient, who has difficulty in accepting a non-physical explanation for the pain.

Other physical causes of headache and facial pain

It is important to remember that pains in the head and face may be non-neurological in nature, and more the province of the GP or other medical or surgical specialist. Some of these conditions are very common. They are listed in Table 3.1.

Table 3.1 Non-neurological causes of headache and facial pain

Eyes
- Eye strain.
- Glaucoma.
- Iritis.

Teeth
- Caries.
- Malocclusion.

Sinuses
- Infection.
- Malignant disease.

Temporo-mandibular joints
- Arthritis.

Ears
- Otitis media and externa.

Heart
- Angina may be felt in the neck and jaws.

Chapter 4

Dementia

Introduction

Dementia, loss of intellectual function, is common in Western society, and it is becoming more common as the age of the population gradually increases. Already patients with dementia are creating a major load upon community and hospital medical services.

The occurrence of dementia is often not too distressing for the patient, who frequently lacks insight, though the consequences for the patient's relatives are usually far-reaching and very disappointing. Asked earlier in their lives, many people would rather die than suffer the humiliation of losing their intellect, becoming 'child-like' or 'senile', dependent on others through inability to think for themselves. In practice, however, a steady enlargement of psycho-geriatric services is occurring to accommodate an increasing number of patients who have lost their memory and intelligence, yet who are otherwise fit and able to survive for many years.

Not all cases of dementia are as gloomy as this in terms of severity, inevitable progression, lack of treatment or need for long-term hospitalization. This will become apparent later in the chapter when individual causes of dementia are discussed.

Before discussing dementia in detail, some attention should be given to two related, but clinically distinct, entities: mental retardation and pseudo-dementia.

Mental retardation

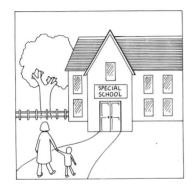

Synonyms for mental retardation include 'a low intelligence quotient', 'mentally backward', 'mentally handicapped', and 'educationally subnormal'. The difference between dementia and mental retardation is that patients with dementia have had normal intelligence in their adult life and then start to lose it, whereas mentally retarded patients have suffered some insult to their brains early in their life which has prevented the development of normal intelligence.

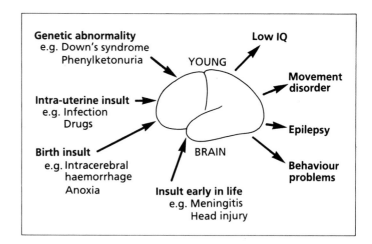

Fig. 4.1. Diagram to show the common insults that can occur to the developing brain, and their consequences.

Whereas dementia is frequently a progressive process, mental retardation is not. The mentally retarded person learns, develops and improves but at a slow rate and to a limited extent, dictated by the fact that the brain is substandard.

A brain that has been damaged in some way early in life may express this damage in any or all of four main ways.

1 Impaired intellectual function, thinking, memory, vocabulary, school work, etc.

2 Impaired movement of the body, because of damage to the parts of the brain involved in movement (motor cortex, basal ganglia, cerebellum, thalamus, sensory cortex). Hence:
- delayed milestones for sitting, crawling, walking;
- infantile hemiplegia;
- diplegia, i.e. double hemiplegia (Little's disease);
- choreo-athetoid movements;
- clumsy, poorly coordinated movement.

3 Epilepsy, the physical damage to the brain created an epileptogenic focus.

4 Behaviour problems because of slowness in learning behavioural customs, control of emotions, and right from wrong.

It is possible to construct a diagram which shows the common sort of insult that may occur to the developing brain and the possible consequences (see Fig. 4.1).

Pseudo-dementia

A few patients may deliberately affect loss of memory and impaired intellectual function. In the main, however, pseudo-dementia refers to the impaired thinking that occurs in some patients with depression. Some severely depressed patients may be mentally and physically retarded to a major

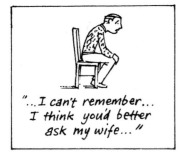

"...I can't remember... I think you'd better ask my wife..."

degree. There may be long intervals between question and answer when interviewing such patients. The patient's feelings of unworthiness and lack of confidence may be such that he is quite uncertain whether his thoughts and answers are accurate or of any value. Patients like this often state quite categorically that they cannot think or remember properly, and defer to their spouse when asked questions. Their overall functional performance, at work or in the house, may become grossly impaired because of mental slowness, indecisiveness, lack of enthusiasm and impaired energy.

> . . . . . a forgetful person, in no real distress, who can no longer do their job, can no longer be independent, and who cannot really sustain any ordinary sensible conversation.

Features of dementia

The commonly encountered defects in intellectual function that occur in patients with dementia, together with the effects that such defects have, are shown below. Because the dementing process usually develops slowly, the features of dementia evolve insidiously, and are often 'absorbed' by the patient's family. This is why the patient may exhibit marked features of intellectual impairment by the time that medical assistance is sought.

Defect in:	Effects:
Memory	• Disorientation, especially in time • Impaired knowledge of recent events • Forgets messages, repeats himself • Loses things about the house • Impaired care of personal cleanliness and appearance • Increasing dependence on familiar surroundings and daily routine
Thinking, understanding, reasoning and initiating	• Poor organization • Ordinary jobs muddled and poorly executed • Slow, inaccurate, circumstantial conversation • Poor comprehension of argument, conversation and TV programmes • Difficulty in making decisions and judgements • Fewer new ideas, less initiative • Increasing dependence on relatives
Dominant hemisphere function	• Reduced vocabulary • Over-use of simple phrases • Reading and writing problems • Spelling problems • Inability to handle money
Non-dominant hemisphere function	• Easily lost • Wandering • Difficulty in dressing
Insight and emotion	• Usually lacking in insight, facile • Occasionally insight is intact, causing anxiety and depression • Emotional lability may be present

Testing intellectual function (with some reference to anatomical localization)

Talking to the patient, in an attempt to obtain details of the history, will have indicated the presence of impairment of intellectual function in most instances. The next tasks are to find out how severely affected intellectual function is, and whether all aspects of the intellect are involved, i.e. global dementia, or whether the problem is localized.

It is important to establish early on in the examination whether there is a significant degree of expressive or receptive dysphasia. If such a defect is present, it is very difficult to proceed with further testing of intellectual function, since one cannot be sure if errors in reply to questions are due to impairment of intellect, or simply due to the impaired receptive or expressive processing of words.

Usually, an expressive dysphasia will have shown itself during the history-taking. Use of wrong words, intervals when the patient has been unable to find the word he wants to use, and frustration over vocabulary will have been apparent. A receptive dysphasia may also have been noticed by virtue of the use of wrong words which the patient does not seem to have noticed. The presence of a receptive dysphasia can be sought quickly, and early, by asking the patient to obey simple (one, two or three component) instructions, e.g. 'lift up your arm'; 'put one hand on your chest and the other on your head'; 'touch your nose, put on your spectacles and stand up'.

If there is no major dysphasic problem, examination of other aspects of intellectual function may proceed.

Whole cerebrum

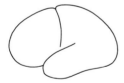

The whole cerebrum, particularly the frontal and temporal regions and the structures around the 3rd ventricle, governs:
- memory;
- thinking;
- concentration;
- attention;
- judgement;
- insight;
- behaviour.

Observations to be made:
- personal appearance, cleanliness, clothes;
- does the patient have insight? is his mood appropriate?
- is he orientated in time, place and person?
- can he retain digits in his head? can he repeat 5 or 6 digits without any pause?

- can he recall a name and address, immediately and after 5 minutes?
- how is his general knowledge for current and for past events? (memory for recent events tends to be lost first in organic dementia).

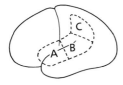

Dominant hemisphere

Spoken language (A)

- Even though there may be no major dysphasic problem, is there some reduction in the patient's vocabulary, some difficulty naming objects in succession, occasional misuse of words or difficulty in word-finding?

Written language (B)

- Are there difficulties in reading (dyslexia), writing (dysgraphia) or calculation (dyscalculia)? These can all be checked at the bedside or in the clinic with paper and pencil.

Parietal lobe dysfunction (C)

- Is there contralateral limb sensory inattention or contralateral homonymous visual field inattention?
- Is there constructional dyspraxia in which the patient has difficulty when asked to draw complex shapes (e.g. a house, a star), or to arrange matchsticks into shapes of this sort?

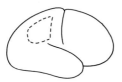

Non-dominant hemisphere

- Is there contralateral limb inattention or visual inattention (which is often marked with non-dominant parietal lobe lesions)?
- Is there spatial disorientation, so that the patient becomes lost in familiar surroundings, has difficulty in locating well-known places on maps, and struggles with correct arrangement of his clothes on his body (dressing dyspraxia)?

Causes of dementia

The commoner causes of organic dementia are listed below, followed by brief notes about each of the individual causes.
1 Alzheimer's disease.
2 Multi-infarct dementia.

3 Other progressive intracranial pathology:
- Parkinson's disease;
- multiple sclerosis;
- cerebral tumour;
- chronic subdural haematoma;
- chronic hydrocephalus;
- Huntington's chorea.

4 As a non-progressive sequel to a single major intracranial disaster:
- head trauma;
- intracranial haemorrhage;
- meningitis; encephalitis; abscess;
- an episode of cerebral anoxia.

5 Alcohol and drugs.

6 Rare infections, deficiencies and metabolic disorders:
- AIDS;
- syphilis;
- Jakob–Creutzfeldt disease;
- B vitamin deficiency;
- hypothyroidism.

Alzheimer's disease

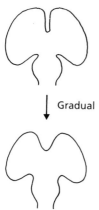

Gradual

This is very common, usually presenting in patients over 50 years of age. There is early and severe involvement of memory. Insight is usually lost. Alzheimer's disease gradually affects all aspects of intellectual function. Epilepsy and focal neurological deficits are very uncommon, and walking is unaffected. The disease, and the dementia it causes, are insidious and patients often present very late.

The main cell loss and morphological change are in the cerebral cortex, but important changes are also present in nuclei in the region of the midbrain and basal ganglia. These more central nuclei, composed of cholinergic neurones, normally project widely to the cerebral cortex, and their loss may be important in the evolution or clinical expression of Alzheimer's disease.

Multi-infarct dementia

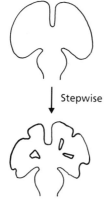

Stepwise

This is common, especially in patients with hypertension and/or evidence of atheroma, i.e. stroke, myocardial infarction, intermittent claudication. It is characterized by episodic, stepwise evolution of dementia rather than an insidiously progressive process.

Focal neurological deficits (e.g. dysphasia, dysarthria, hemiparesis, visual field defect, ataxia) are common in the history and on examination. Walking is frequently abnormal because of hemiparesis or ataxia, or because of the development of a rather complex gait disturbance, consisting of small shuffling steps (*marche à petit pas*). Emotional lability is often conspicuous, along with other evidence of pseudobulbar palsy (brisk jaw-jerk and spastic dysarthria).

Multiple infarcts of different sizes are found throughout all parts of the brain.

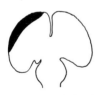

Chronic subdural
haematoma

Other progressive intracranial pathology

Dementia may be a feature in patients who have either Parkinson's disease or multiple sclerosis very severely. In such cases, there is no doubt of the cause of the dementia (because the primary condition is so severe). Allowance must be made for its presence when discussing drug treatment and management.

Frontal and temporal lobe tumours may cause significant impairment of intellectual function before producing telltale features of a focal neurological deficit or raised intracranial pressure. Patients with chronic subdural haematoma are usually elderly or alcoholic. Their dementia is usually associated with drowsiness and evolves in a few weeks. Any process which causes hydrocephalus slowly may declare itself by failing intellectual ability, slowness and drowsiness, often with headaches and gait unsteadiness.

Dementia is an early feature of the clinical presentation of Huntington's chorea. Dementia is frequently a major problem in patient management in this condition, and the reason for eventual institutionalization. There will usually be a positive family history.

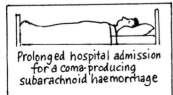

Prolonged hospital admission
for a coma-producing
subarachnoid haemorrhage

Non-progressive sequel to a major intracranial disaster

After any of the conditions mentioned under this category in the list above, organic dementia may be one of the residual deficits. Other neurological abnormalities are likely. A coexistent depression is also likely if insight is preserved in such circumstances. Staff working in rehabilitation units are skilled in evaluating intellectual function in such patients, and often provide a very favourable environment for optimization of recovery.

Alcohol and drugs

In addition to the rather flamboyant syndromes seen in alcoholics who become deficient in vitamin B_1, namely Wernicke's encephalopathy and Korsakoff's psychosis, it is being increasingly recognized that chronic alcoholism is associated with cerebral atrophy and generalized dementia.

Patients, especially those who are elderly, may become confused and forgetful whilst on medication, especially antidepressants, tranquillizers, hypnotics, analgesics and anticonvulsants.

It is most important to bear in mind alcohol and drugs before embarking upon a detailed investigation of dementia.

Rare infections, deficiencies and metabolic disorders

AIDS

It is becoming increasingly evident that patients with AIDS undergo a slow dementing process, which is due to the human immuno-deficiency virus' presence in the brain causing a low-grade encephalitis. This is a separate process to the effects of opportunistic CNS infections and unusual brain tumours which may develop in AIDS patients.

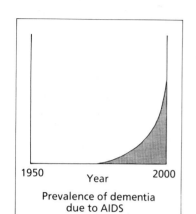

Prevalence of dementia
due to AIDS

Tertiary syphilis

Tertiary syphilis, giving rise to general paralysis of the insane, tabes dorsalis, tabo-paresis (features of both of the former) and meningovascular syphilis, are all extremely rare in civilized societies now due to the common use of penicillin, which is lethal to the spirochaete, *Treponema pallidum*. Any patient whose dementia is associated with abnormal neurological signs should prompt the possibility of neurosyphilis in the doctor's mind, especially if the pupils are abnormal, the knee or ankle jerks absent, or the plantar responses extensor. Marked frontal lobe features in the dementia, e.g. grandiose ideas or behaviour, and antisocial behaviour, should trigger the possibility of this diagnosis in the doctor's mind also.

Jakob–Creutzfeldt disease

Jakob–Creutzfeldt disease usually produces a rapidly progressive neurological degenerative disease in which dementia is associated with physical disability, to render the patient bed-bound and helpless within months. Myoclonic jerks occur in the process of this illness. It is extremely rare but important to remember because of its transmissibility. Though an infective agent has not been positively identified in the brains of patients with this condition, innoculation of primate's brain with brain tissue from affected patients will establish the same condition in the primate some 1–2 years later.

B vitamin deficiency

Vitamin B₁ deficiency in Western society occurs in alcoholics whose diet is inadequate, and in people who voluntarily modify their diet to an extreme degree, e.g. patients with anorexia nervosa or extreme vegetarians.

Impairment of short-term memory, drowsiness, abnormalities of eye movement and pupils, together with ataxia, constitute the features of Wernicke's encephalopathy. Though associated with demonstrable pathology in the midbrain, this syndrome is often rapidly reversible by urgent thiamine replacement.

Less reversible is the chronic state of short-term memory impairment and confabulation which characterize Korsakoff's psychosis, mainly seen in advanced alcoholism.

Whether *vitamin B₁₂ deficiency* causes dementia remains uncertain. Certainly, peripheral neuropathy and subacute combined degeneration of the spinal cord are more definite neurological consequences of deficiency in this vitamin.

Hypothyroidism

Hypothyroidism is usually rather evident clinically by the time significant impairment of intellectual function is present. It is a cause worth remembering in view of its obvious reversibility.

Investigation of dementia

Very frequently, an accurate history, together with a full physical examination, will have highlighted the most likely cause for an individual patient's dementia.

The services of a clinical psychologist may be very useful in assessing the degree and breadth of loss of intellectual function, and in commenting upon insight and depression.

Particular tests that may be important include:

- blood: Hb, MCV;
  LFTs (including gamma GT);
  serological tests for syphilis;
  serological tests for AIDS;
  drug levels;
  B_{12};
  thyroid function tests;
- CT brain scan;
- CSF analysis (including tests for syphilis);
- chest X-ray and ECG.

Management of dementia

Careful explanation is important, mainly to the family of the demented person. Clearly, any treatable condition will be treated, but most usually it is necessary to explain that there is not any specific treatment for the patient's dementia. The family must be helped to realize that the demented patient will continue to be dependent on them, will thrive better on a regular routine each day, and may need a certain amount of custodial care to prevent danger from fire, electricity, etc. around the home. Night sedation may be necessary. In more severely affected cases, help and relief in the form of somebody sitting with the patient whilst relatives shop or pursue some recreation, or in the form of day-centre attendance, may be required. If the dementia is very severe or supportive relatives are not available, the patient may require permanent institutionalization.

It may be necessary to encourage the healthy spouse to seek power of attorney, and to obtain advice regarding pensions, investments, and wills from a solicitor.

Chapter 5

Scheme for understanding disorders of movement

This is a short chapter, which is set out very diagrammatically, with three aims in mind:

1 to remind the reader of the various components of the nervous system which are involved in normal movement;

2 to characterize the kind of movement abnormality that occurs when each of these individual components is not working properly;

3 to mention the common clinical patterns and syndromes of movement disorder.

This is done at a simple, rather naive, level to provide a clear introductory framework for understanding the disorders of movement described in subsequent chapters.

Basic components of the nervous system required for normal movement

Lesions along the primary motor pathway, UMN–LMN–NMJ–M, are characterized by weakness or paralysis. The characteristics of the weakness are different in each instance, for instance UMN weakness has different characteristics to LMN weakness. Knowledge of these characteristics is fundamental to clinical neurology.

Normal cerebellar, basal ganglion and sensory function is essential background activity of the nervous system for normal movement. Lesions in these parts of the nervous system do not produce weakness or paralysis, but make movement imperfect because of clumsiness, stiffness, slowness, involuntary movement or lack of adequate feeling.

UMN = Upper motor neurone
LMN = Lower motor neurone
NMJ = Neuromuscular junction
M = Muscle
C = Cerebellum
BG = Basal ganglia
S = Sensation

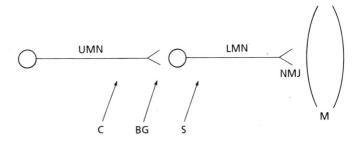

Upper motor neurone

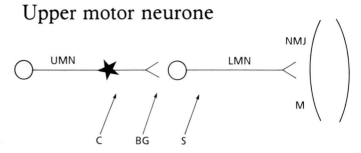

Characteristics of upper motor neurone lesions:
- no wasting;
- increased tone of clasp-knife type;
- weakness most evident in anti-gravity muscles;
- increased reflexes and clonus;
- extensor plantar responses.

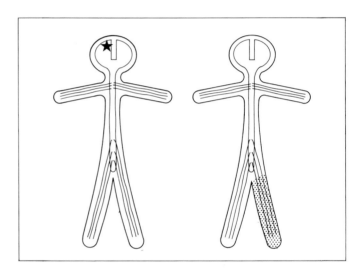

Contralateral monoparesis
A lesion situated peripherally in the cerebral hemisphere, i.e. involving part of the motor homunculus only, produces weakness of part of the contralateral side of the body, e.g. the contralateral leg. If the lesion also involves the adjacent sensory homunculus in the post-central gyrus, there may be some sensory loss in the same part of the body.

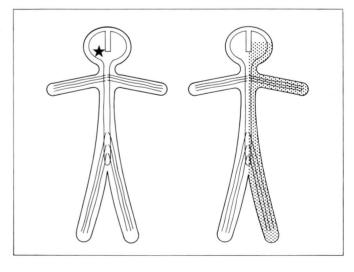

Contralateral hemiparesis
Lesions situated deep in the cerebral hemisphere, in the region of the internal capsule, are much more likely to produce weakness of the whole of the contralateral side of the body, face, arm and leg. Because of the condensation of fibre pathways in the region of the internal capsule, such lesions commonly produce significant contralateral sensory loss (hemianaesthesia) and visual loss (homonymous hemianopia), in addition to the hemiparesis.

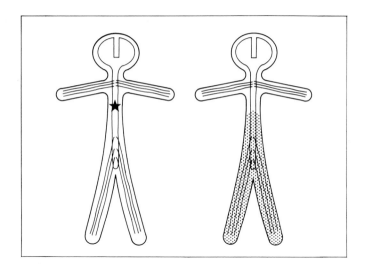

Paraparesis
UMN weakness of the legs occurs with lesions situated at or below the cervical portion of the spinal cord.

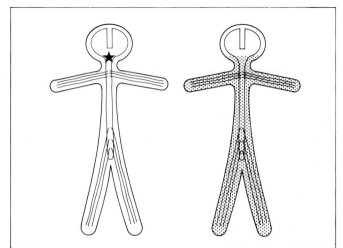

Quadriparesis or tetraparesis
UMN weakness of all four limbs occurs with lesions which are situated in the midbrain, pons, brainstem, and upper cervical cord.

Lesions anywhere between midbrain and lower spinal cord may, in addition, involve ascending sensory pathways and fibre tracts involving sphincter function. There may therefore be sensory loss below the level of the lesion, and the possibility of bladder, bowel and sexual symptoms.

There may be physical signs which indicate the level of the lesion very accurately:

• LMN signs, loss of reflexes, dermatome pain, or sensory loss, at the level of the lesion in the spinal cord;
• cerebellar signs or cranial nerve palsies when the lesion is in the midbrain, pons or medulla.

Lower motor neurone

NMJ

UMN ⟨ LMN ★ ⟨

M

C BG S

Characteristics of lower motor neurone lesions:
- wasting;
- fasciculation;
- decreased tone (i.e. flaccidity);
- weakness;
- decreased or absent reflexes;
- flexor or absent plantar responses.

Generalized LMN weakness may result from pathology affecting the LMNs throughout the spinal cord and brainstem, as in motor neurone disease or poliomyelitis. Generalized limb weakness (proximal and distal), trunk and bulbar weakness characterize this sort of LMN disorder.

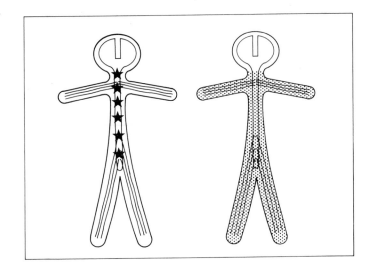

Generalized LMN weakness may also result from widespread damage to the axons of the LMNs. This is the nature of peripheral neuropathy (also called polyneuropathy). The axons of the dorsal root sensory neurones are usually simultaneously involved. The LMN weakness and sensory loss tend to be most marked distally in the limbs.

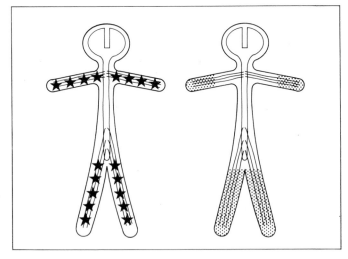

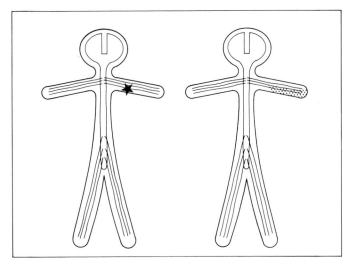

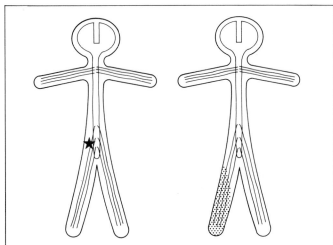

LMN weakness may be confined to the distribution of one peripheral nerve (*above*) or one spinal nerve root (*below*). In such circumstances, the LMN signs are found only in the distribution of the particular nerve or nerve root in question, and almost always there is sensory impairment or loss in the area supplied by the nerve or nerve root. Examples of such lesions are an ulnar nerve lesion at the elbow, or an L5 nerve root syndrome caused by a prolapsed intervertebral disc.

Neuromuscular junction

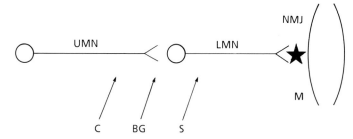

Characteristics of myasthenia gravis:
- uncommon;
- no wasting;
- tone normal;
- weakness;
- fatiguability;
- reflexes normal;
- positive response to anticholinesterase.

The pattern of muscle involvement in this rare disease:
- ocular muscles common:
  ptosis;
  diplopia;
- bulbar muscles fairly common:
  dysarthria;
  dysphagia;
- trunk and limb muscles less common:
  limb weakness;
  trunk weakness;
  breathing problems.

More common paralysis due to neuromuscular blockade is that which is produced by anaesthetists during operative surgery.

Muscle

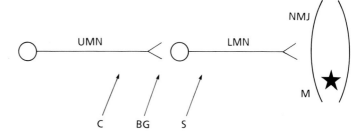

Characteristics of primary muscle disease:
- uncommon;
- wasting;
- no fasciculation;
- weakness;
- tone normal or reduced;
- reflexes normal or reduced.

Pattern of muscle involvement:
- specific in familial muscular dystrophies, e.g. facio-scapulo-humeral;
- proximal weakness in the limbs in the acquired diseases of muscle, e.g. polymyositis.

Cerebellum

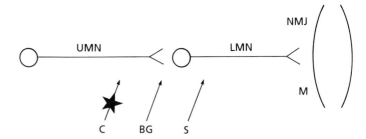

Characteristics of cerebellar lesions:
- incoordination of muscle activity:

  in cranial nerve territory: nystagmus, dysarthria

  in the arms: finger–nose ataxia, intention tremor, dysdiadokokinesia

  in the legs: heel–knee–shin ataxia, gait ataxia, falls
- in a unilateral cerebellar lesion, the neurological deficit is ipsilateral to the side of the lesion;
- there is no weakness. (Alcohol in large doses impairs cerebellar function. Intoxicated people show all the features of muscular incoordination mentioned above, but may be very strong.)

Basal ganglia

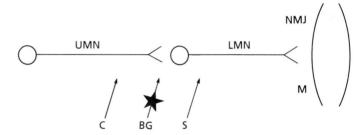

Two main syndromes, each with different characteristics:
1 Parkinson's disease:
 • common;
 • tremor at rest;
 • increased tone;
 • bradykinesia;
 • posture of universal flexion;
2 Choreo-athetoid syndromes:
 • uncommon;
 • involuntary movements at rest and during action;
 • tone increased, normal or reduced;
 • normal speed of movement;
 • all sorts of postural abnormalities;
No weakness in either.

These syndromes may be unilateral and are commonly
asymmetrical, the pathology being in the basal ganglia in
the contralateral cerebral hemisphere.

Sensation

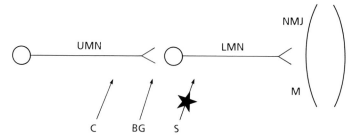

Characteristics of movement in the presence of sensory loss:
- ataxia or clumsiness of movement due to loss of sense of position mainly, but also due to loss of touch sensation;
- partial compensation by active monitoring of movement by the eyes;
- no weakness.

Two clinical situations where sensory loss may play an important role in impairing movement:

1 peripheral neuropathy:
- impaired manipulation of objects in numb fingers which lack proprioception;
- impaired balance on numb feet which lack proprioception;

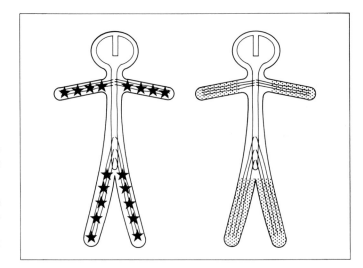

2 cerebral hemisphere lesion:
- impaired accurate movement of the contralateral limbs when central registration of limb position is lost.

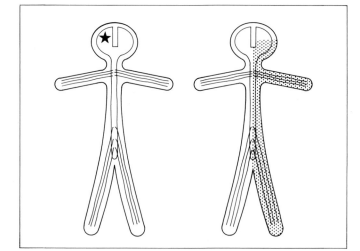

Chapter 6   Stroke

Introduction

Cerebrovascular disease is common, especially in Western civilized countries where an increasing proportion of people survive to old age. All forms of cerebrovascular disease are more common in patients with hypertension. Cerebrovascular disease is responsible, therefore, for considerable mortality, and it is a major cause of disability, especially in the elderly and hypertensive.

Sudden loss of neurological function is the hallmark of cerebrovascular disease. Despite the efforts of preventive medicine, it is frequent for the episode to occur unannounced. In most patients, therefore, the aims of the medical and paramedical professions are twofold:
1 to optimize recovery from the unannounced episode;
2 to prevent the occurrence of further similar events.

Cerebral ischaemia and infarction

Anatomy and pathology

The principal pathological process under consideration here is the occlusion of arteries supplying the brain. The two internal carotid arteries and the basilar artery form the Circle of Willis at the base of the brain, which acts as an efficient anastomotic device in the event of occlusion of arteries proximal to it (i.e. either internal carotid artery or either vertebral artery in the neck) (see Fig. 6.1).

The branches from the Circle of Willis, i.e. the anterior, middle and posterior cerebral arteries supplying the cerebrum, and the branches of the vertebral and basilar arteries directly supplying the brainstem and cerebellum, are all essentially end-arteries, with poorly evolved anastomoses with arteries supplying adjacent territory. Restoration of normal perfusion in tissue made ischaemic by occlusion of one of these end-arteries cannot rely on blood reaching the ischaemic area through anastomotic channels. Recovery of function in the ischaemic tissue depends much more upon

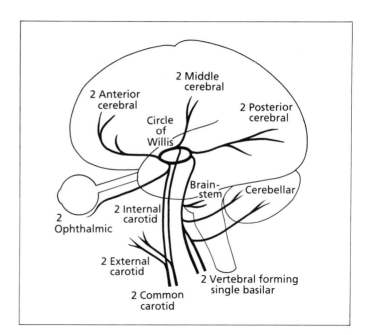

Fig. 6.1. A schematic diagram of the arteries supplying the brain.

lysis or fragmentation of the occluding thrombo-embolic material.

Three other points are worth noting.

1 The ophthalmic arteries are derived from the internal carotid arteries just below the Circle of Willis. They form good anastomotic connections with branches of the external carotid arteries in the orbits, and they sometimes provide an effective way for blood to reach the brain when the internal carotid arteries are narrowed or occluded in the neck.

2 The middle cerebral arteries are the largest of the branches from the Circle of Willis, so that any embolic material arriving at the Circle of Willis is more likely to find its way into these arteries. Brain tissue supplied by the middle cerebral arteries is frequently involved in patients presenting with cerebral ischaemia or infarction.

3 Though the vertebral arteries arrive at the skull base in a most unusual way, through a series of foramina in the transverse processes of the cervical vertebrae, they are not easily compressed by head and neck movements, even in the presence of cervical disc degenerative disease.

Occlusion of one of the cerebral arteries may result from local thrombus formation in the artery at the site of local atheroma. More commonly, occlusion is caused by embolic material derived either from the heart, or from thrombus associated with atheroma in the aorta or major arteries in the neck. Occlusion leads to sudden severe ischaemia in the area of brain tissue supplied by the occluded artery, and recovery depends upon rapid lysis or fragmentation of the occluding material. Reversal of neurological function within minutes or hours gives rise to the clinical picture of a *transient ischaemic attack*. When the neurological deficit lasts longer than 24 hours, it may be called a *reversible ischaemic neurological deficit* if it recovers completely in a few days, or a *completed stroke* if there is a persistent deficit. Sometimes recovery is very slow and incomplete.

Neurological symptoms and signs

The loss of function that the patient notices, and which may be apparent on examination, entirely depends on the area of brain tissue involved in the ischaemic process, as shown in Fig. 6.2.

The following suggest *middle cerebral territory:*
- dysphasia;
- dyslexia, dysgraphia, dyscalculia;
- loss of use of contralateral face and arm;
- loss of feeling in contralateral face and arm.

The following suggests *anterior cerebral territory:*
- loss of use and/or feeling in the contralateral leg.

Fig. 6.2. Arterial territories and localization of function within the brain.

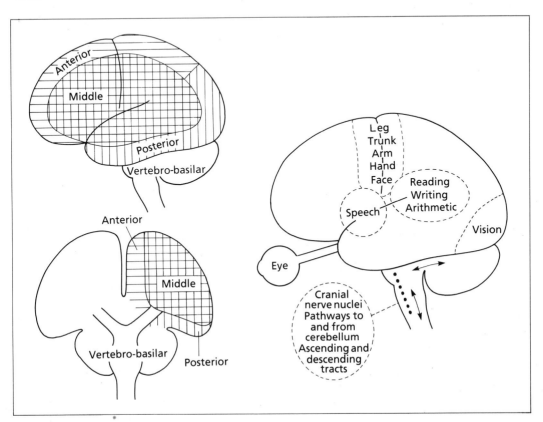

The following suggests *posterior cerebral territory:*
- development of a contralateral homonymous hemianopia.

The following suggests a deep-seated lesion affecting the internal capsule which is supplied by *small perforating branches of the middle and posterior cerebral arteries* close to their origins:
- complete loss of motor and sensory function throughout the whole of the contralateral side of the body with a homonymous hemianopia.

The following suggests *ophthalmic artery territory* (the ophthalmic artery arises from the internal carotid artery just below the Circle of Willis):
- monocular loss of vision.

The following suggest *vertebro-basilar territory:*
- double vision (3, 4, 6);
- facial numbness (5);
- facial weakness (7);
- vertigo (8);
- dysphagia (9, 10);
- dysarthria (9, 10, 12);
- ataxia;
- drop attacks;
- motor or sensory loss in *both* arms or legs.

Symptoms and signs of the cause

The common conditions which give rise to cerebral ischaemia and infarction are listed below.

1 *Cardiac disease* associated with embolization:
- atrial fibrillation;
- mural thrombosis after myocardial infarction;
- aortic or mitral valve disease;
- subacute bacterial endocarditis.

2 *Atheroma* either in the large neck arteries or in the cerebral arteries close to the brain.

There may be a history of other evidence of atheroma:
- previous heart attack;
- angina pectoris;
- intermittent claudication in the legs;
- previous transient ischaemic attacks or stroke.

Bruits may be heard over the carotid, subclavian, or femoral arteries. Leg pulses may be absent.

There may be evidence of conditions known to predispose to atheroma:

- hypertension;
- diabetes;
- hyperlipidaemia;
- smoking;
- obesity.

Less common conditions associated with cerebral ischaemia and infarction are as follows.

1 *Unusual cardiac conditions* giving rise to emboli:
- non-bacterial endocarditis;
- atrial myxoma;
- mitral valve prolapse;
- paradoxical embolization in the presence of a right to left shunt in the heart.

2 *Unusual embolic material:*
- fat;
- air.

3 *Increased blood viscosity:*
- dehydration;
- polycythaemia;
- macroglobulinaemia.

4 *Non-atheromatous arterial disease* predisposing to occlusion and thrombus formation:
- giant cell arteritis;
- collagen vascular disease.

5 *Venous infarction*, in which there is lack of perfusion of brain tissue drained by compressed, infected or thrombosed veins:
- sagittal sinus thrombosis;
- cortical thrombophlebitis.

Management of cerebral ischaemia and infarction

There are two aspects of management, which are carried out simultaneously.

Optimization of recovery from the current neurological deficit

The keys to success in this aspect are:
- careful explanation to, and encouragement of, the patient and his relatives;
- early mobilization to prevent the secondary problems of pneumonia, deep vein thrombosis, pulmonary embolism, pressure sores, frozen shoulder and contractures;
- early socialization to help to prevent depression, and help the acceptance of any disability;
- maintenance of a good blood pressure over the first few weeks, avoiding over-enthusiastic treatment of hypertension

(cerebral perfusion in the ischaemic area is very dependent on blood pressure, because of impaired autoregulation);
- early involvement of physiotherapists, speech therapists and occupational therapists, as necessary. Provision of simple aids and gadgets;
- consideration of involvement of a local rehabilitation unit;
- attention to occupational and financial consequences of the event, with the help of a medical social worker if appropriate.

Prevention of further similar episodes

This means the identification and treatment of the aetiological factors already mentioned.

Careful clinical examination of the patient, quite apart from neurological examination, is important therefore and should involve:
- checking the cardiac rhythm;
- measuring the blood pressure;
- listening to the heart;
- checking all the peripheral pulses;
- listening to the carotid, subclavian and femoral arteries;
- noting the patient's weight, exercise and smoking habits;
- checking for glycosuria.

The search for any causative factors is extended by investigation:
- Hb, PCV, WCC, platelets, ESR;
- chest X-ray;
- ECG;
- fasting blood glucose;
- fasting blood lipids;
- cardiological investigation if there is any indication of embolization from the heart.

If there is strong evidence of ipsilateral carotid artery disease, further investigation may be embarked upon to demonstrate this. Several non-invasive techniques are available, though angiography remains the most reliable to date. Angiography, which involves arterial puncture, carries some risk, and should be carried out only if there is a definite intention to proceed to carotid artery endarterectomy if appropriate atheromatous disease is shown. The benefits of such surgery are yet to be clearly established.

Where no factors of aetiological significance can be established, there may be little that can be done to prevent subsequent similar episodes. Agents that reduce platelet adhesiveness have been shown to reduce slightly the incidence of non-fatal and fatal stroke, and of myocardial infarction, in patients with a history of transient ischaemic attacks or stroke. Formal anticoagulation with warfarin-like drugs has not been shown to be of advantage, except where a cardiac source for embolization has been proved.

In patients in whom further strokes cannot be prevented, an accumulated clinical picture may sometimes evolve. This is not inevitable. When it does occur:
• it may be dominated by impaired intellectual function (so called multi-infarct dementia, described in Chapter 4);
• it may be more a matter of several physical deficits affecting vision, speech, limb movement and balance. Some degree of pseudo-bulbar palsy (with slurred speech, brisk jaw-jerk and emotional lability) is common in such cases due to the bilateral cerebral hemisphere involvement, affecting upper motor neurone innervation of the lower cranial nerve nuclei;
• the diffuse ischaemic change may show itself in the patient's gait, causing the *marche à petit pas* (walking by means of minute shuffling steps, which may be out of proportion to the relatively minor abnormal neurological signs to be found in the legs on formal examination).

Subarachnoid haemorrhage and intracerebral haemorrhage

Anatomy and pathology

The pathological process here is the sudden release of arterial blood, either into the subarachnoid space around the brain, or directly into the substance of the brain. In the case of subarachnoid haemorrhage, the bleeding usually occurs from berry aneurysms located on the arteries at the base of the brain, close to the arterial Circle of Willis (Fig. 6.3, *left*). Intracerebral haemorrhage most frequently occurs in the presence of arterial hypertension, from very small micro-aneurysms on long thin penetrating arteries in critically important regions of the brain, the internal capsule or the pons (Fig. 6.3, *right*). Arterio-venous malformations oc-casionally occur in the head, and are capable of bleeding into the subarachnoid space or into the substance of the brain. They are rare.

Both subarachnoid haemorrhage and intracerebral haem-orrhage are much more destructive and dangerous con-ditions than ischaemic cerebrovascular disease. A proportion of patients with either of these two conditions die within hours or days of the haemorrhage. In the case of subarachnoid haemorrhage, there is a definite risk of re-bleeding in a patient surviving the first bleed from the

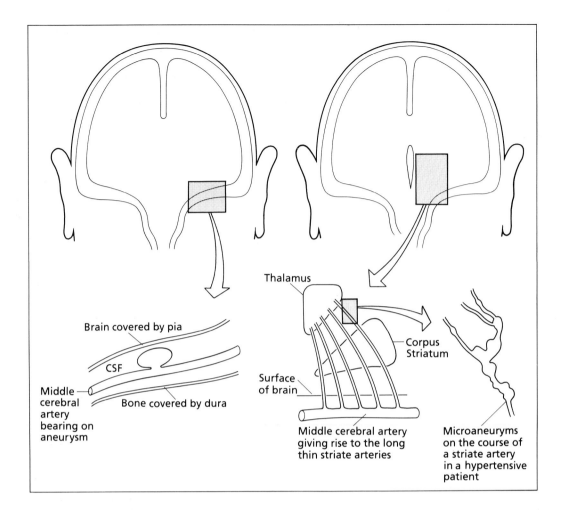

Thalamus

Brain covered by pia

CSF

Corpus
Striatum

Middle
cerebral
artery
bearing on
aneurysm

Bone covered by dura

Surface
of brain

Middle cerebral artery
giving rise to the long
thin striate arteries

Microaneuryms
on the course of
a striate artery
in a hypertensive
patient

Fig. 6.3. *Left:* Berry aneurysm, the common cause of subarachnoid haemorrhage. *Right:* Micro-aneurysms, the common cause of intracerebral haemorrhage.

aneurysm. There is a higher incidence of severe neurological deficit in patients surviving subarachnoid or intracerebral haemorrhage compared with those surviving episodes of cerebral ischaemia or infarction. Subarachnoid and intracerebral haemorrhage are less common than cerebral ischaemia or infarction. We should have the concept, therefore, of intracranial haemorrhage being an occasional, severe condition with high mortality and morbidity, and occlusive cerebrovascular disease as a more common condition with a far wider range of severity.

Neurological symptoms and signs

Subarachnoid haemorrhage from a berry aneurysm on or near the Circle of Willis can produce a variety of consequences, as shown in Fig. 6.4.

Figure 6.5 shows the sites and effects of intracerebral haemorrhage.

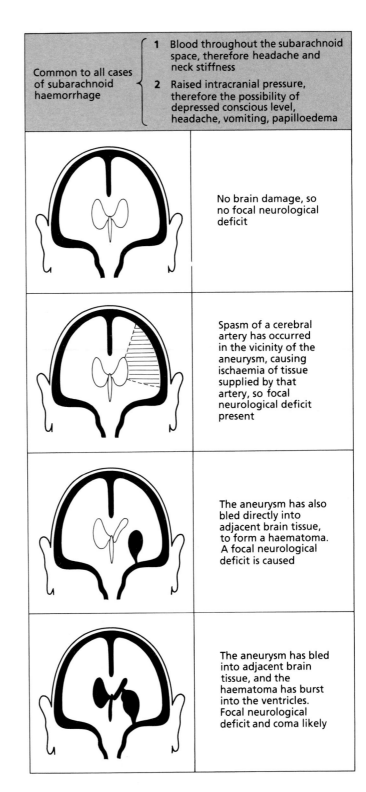

Fig. 6.4. Diagram to show the clinical features of subarachnoid haemorrhage.

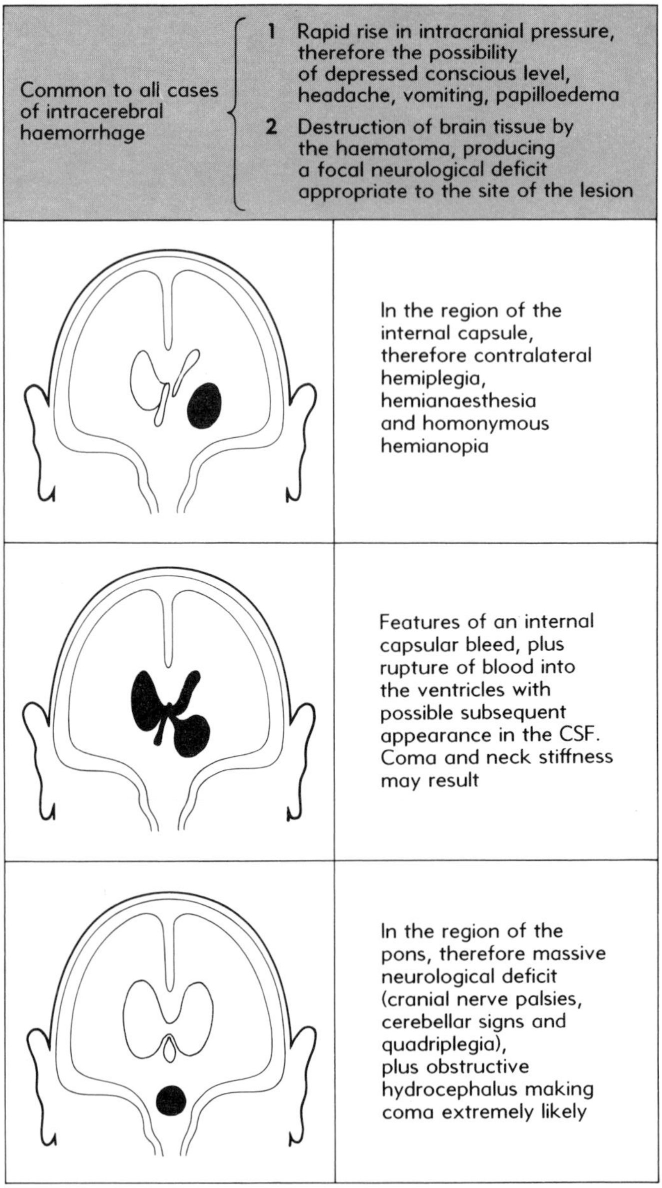

| Common to all cases of intracerebral haemorrhage | 1 Rapid rise in intracranial pressure, therefore the possibility of depressed conscious level, headache, vomiting, papilloedema |
| | 2 Destruction of brain tissue by the haematoma, producing a focal neurological deficit appropriate to the site of the lesion |

In the region of the internal capsule, therefore contralateral hemiplegia, hemianaesthesia and homonymous hemianopia

Features of an internal capsular bleed, plus rupture of blood into the ventricles with possible subsequent appearance in the CSF. Coma and neck stiffness may result

In the region of the pons, therefore massive neurological deficit (cranial nerve palsies, cerebellar signs and quadriplegia), plus obstructive hydrocephalus making coma extremely likely

Fig. 6.5. Diagram to show the clinical features of intracerebral haemorrhage.

It is possible to construct a scheme for understanding the clinical features of subarachnoid haemorrhage and intracerebral haemorrhage as follows.

Both conditions involve the liberation of a volume of arterial blood into the head, which means a sudden rise in intracranial pressure. The features of raised intracranial pressure are:

• a decrease in conscious level;
• headache;
• vomiting;
• papilloedema.

The rapid development of some or all of these features within a minute or two is highly suggestive of an intracranial bleed. Sometimes, the sudden rise in intracranial pressure is so marked that haemorrhage occurs into the retina, or just in front of the retina (subhyaloid haemorrhage).

In *subarachnoid haemorrhage* there is blood throughout the subarachnoid space and blood irritates the meninges. Severe headache and neck stiffness of sudden onset characterize subarachnoid haemorrhage. An immediate focal neurological deficit probably indicates that an associated intracerebral haematoma has formed. A neurological deficit appearing a few days later is more characteristic of associated arterial spasm causing cerebral ischaemia or infarction.

An *intracerebral bleed* in the region of the internal capsule will cause sudden severe motor, sensory and visual problems on the contralateral side of the body (hemiplegia, hemi-anaesthesia and homonymous hemianopia). In the region of the pons, sudden loss of motor and sensory function in all four limbs, associated with disordered brainstem function, accounts for the extremely high mortality of haemorrhage in this area.

Bleeding into the ventricular system, whether the initial bleed is subarachnoid or intracerebral, is of grave prognostic significance. It is frequently found in patients dying within hours of the bleed.

Blood pressure

Any patient who has recently had an intracranial haemorrhage of any sort may show significant transient elevation of blood pressure as a consequence of the bleed. Hypertension proper is more common in patients with subarachnoid haemorrhage than the normal population. Hypertension proper is extremely common in patients with intracerebral haemorrhage. Intracerebral haemorrhage is one of the major complications of untreated hypertension. It is one of the natural causes of death in patients with untreated hypertension.

High blood pressure readings found in patients shortly after a subarachnoid or intracerebral bleed should not automatically lead to over-enthusiastic pharmacological treatment. As in ischaemic stroke, the damaged brain tissue needs a good perfusion pressure to maintain good blood flow rates. Such brain tissue has lost its ability to autoregulate, i.e. to keep a constant blood flow rate despite varying blood pressure levels (which is characteristic of healthy brain tissue). Low blood pressure therefore leads to low blood flow in the recently damaged areas of brain.

Management of subarachnoid haemorrhage

Establish the diagnosis

If there is a typical history, marked neck stiffness and no focal neurological deficit, lumbar puncture is still the best way to make the diagnosis, revealing uniformly blood-stained CSF. If the history is typical with marked neck stiffness, but the patient remains in coma or shows a marked focal neurological deficit, a CT scan is a safer way to establish the diagnosis (revealing blood in the subarachnoid space), since lumbar puncture may lead to coning in this group of patients (whose coma or focal neurological deficit may indicate the presence of an associated intracerebral blood clot).

Prevent re-bleeding

Advice from specialist neurosurgical units should be sought. Patients who have withstood their first bleed well are submitted to carotid and vertebral angiography within a few days to establish whether or not an operable aneurysm is present. Patients who do not recover from their first bleed well, patients with no detectable aneurysm at angiography, and patients with inoperable aneurysms should be nursed in bed for a few weeks and then mobilized over a further few weeks, being encouraged to return to full normal activities at about 3–4 months.

Rehabilitation

Since the incidence of significant damage to the brain is high in patients surviving subarachnoid haemorrhage, many will not be able to return to normal activities. They will need support from relatives, nurses, physiotherapists, speech therapists, occupational therapists, social workers and specialist units in rehabilitation.

Management of intracerebral haemorrhage

Lesions in the pons

The mortality and morbidity of lesions in the pons is such as to make active treatment of any sort of questionable medical or ethical merit.

Lesions in the internal capsule

1 Reduce the damaging effects of the mass lesion (haematoma and surrounding brain oedema) by use of steroids. Occasionally, consideration is given to removing the haematoma if the mass effects are still evident after 7–10 days and the haematoma is large and fairly laterally situated.

2 Attend to the patient's hypertension, gently initially, energetically after a few weeks.

3 Rehabilitation: a major and persistent neurological deficit is to be expected, and all the agencies mentioned under rehabilitation of patients with subarachnoid haemorrhage are likely to be of value.

The *ideal treatment of intracerebral haemorrhage is prophylactic.* There is good evidence to show that conscientious treatment of high blood pressure reduces the incidence of intracerebral haemorrhage in hypertensive patients.

Chapter 7

Brain tumour

Introduction

Like malignant neoplasms anywhere else in the body, histologically malignant brain tumours carry a poor prognosis. Histologically benign brain tumours are often difficult to remove. This may be the result of a lack of clear boundary between tumour tissue and normal brain substance, e.g. a low-grade astrocytoma within the cerebrum. Alternatively, the surgical difficulty may be because the tumour lies very close to a part of the brain with important functions, e.g. a meningioma adjacent to the motor cortex, or an acoustic neuroma lying beside the brainstem.

Brain tumours therefore have an unfavourable reputation. The poor outlook that accompanies brain tumours is all the more frustrating in view of the much improved technology (e.g. computerized tomography and magnetic resonance) used in their detection.

Intracranial compartments, shift, tentorial herniation, coning, lethal lumbar puncture, and false localizing signs

Figure 7.1 shows the rigid frame that contains the brain. The dura lining the inner aspect of the skull, the falx cerebri and the tentorium cerebelli divide the space within the skull into three large compartments. These compartments contain one cerebral hemisphere each above the tentorium cerebelli, and the cerebellum and brainstem in the posterior fossa beneath the tentorium cerebelli. The midbrain passes through the hole in the tentorium, the tentorial hiatus, and the junctional area between the medulla oblongata and the spinal cord occupies the foramen magnum at the bottom of the posterior fossa. Figure 7.1 also shows the ventricular system. Cerebrospinal fluid, produced by the choroid plexus in each of the ventricles, runs downwards through the ventricular system and exits the 4th ventricle to gain the subarachnoid space via the foramina of Luschka and Magendie.

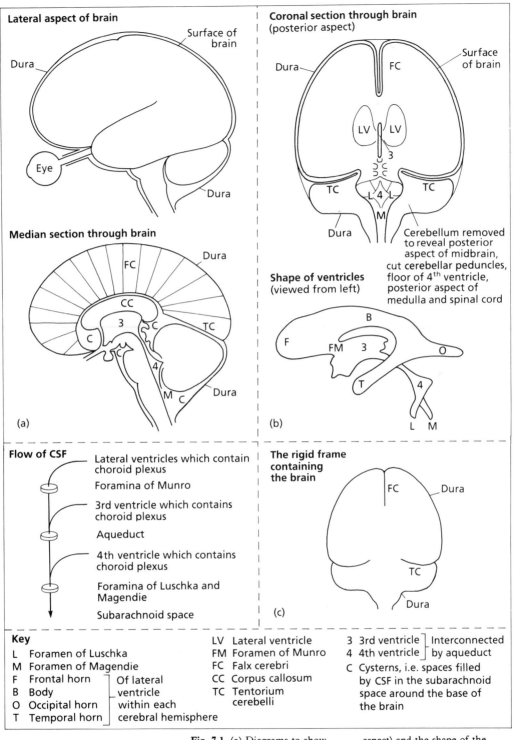

Lateral aspect of brain

Dura

Surface of brain

Eye

Dura

Median section through brain

Dura

FC

CC

3

C

C

TC

4

M

C

Dura

(a)

Coronal section through brain
(posterior aspect)

Dura

FC

Surface of brain

LV

LV

3

TC

TC

L 4 L

M

Dura

Cerebellum removed to reveal posterior aspect of midbrain, cut cerebellar peduncles, floor of 4th ventricle, posterior aspect of medulla and spinal cord

Shape of ventricles
(viewed from left)

B

F

FM

3

O

T

4

L   M

(b)

Flow of CSF

Lateral ventricles which contain choroid plexus

Foramina of Munro

3rd ventricle which contains choroid plexus

Aqueduct

4th ventricle which contains choroid plexus

Foramina of Luschka and Magendie

Subarachnoid space

The rigid frame containing the brain

FC

Dura

TC

Dura

(c)

Key

L	Foramen of Luschka	
M	Foramen of Magendie	
F	Frontal horn ⎤	Of lateral
B	Body	ventricle
O	Occipital horn	within each
T	Temporal horn ⎦	cerebral hemisphere

LV Lateral ventricle
FM Foramen of Munro
FC Falx cerebri
CC Corpus callosum
TC Tentorium cerebelli

3 3rd ventricle ⎤ Interconnected
4 4th ventricle ⎦ by aqueduct
C Cysterns, i.e. spaces filled by CSF in the subarachnoid space around the base of the brain

Fig. 7.1. (a) Diagrams to show the lateral aspect of, and a median section through, the brain. (b) Diagrams to show a coronal section through the brain (posterior aspect) and the shape of the ventricles as viewed from the left. (c) Diagram to show the rigid frame containing the brain.

Figure 7.2 shows the influence of mass lesions situated in different parts of the compartmentalized space within the skull.

When a mass lesion is making one cerebral hemisphere too large for its compartment (Fig. 7.2a):
• the supratentorial midline structures (corpus callosum and 3rd ventricle) are pushed towards the opposite side of the skull below the falx;
• the infero-medial part of the cerebral hemisphere is pushed through the tentorial hiatus (compressing the mid-brain);
• the whole of the brainstem tends to become pushed downwards so that the lowermost parts of the cerebellum and medulla oblongata become impacted in the foramen magnum.

The movement at the tentorial hiatus is known as *tentorial herniation*, and the impaction at the foramen magnum is known as *coning of the medulla*. They commonly occur simultaneously. The effects on the patient are:
• depression in conscious level (due to distortion of the reticular formation lying throughout the whole of the brainstem);
• an impairment of ipsilateral 3rd nerve function, dilatation of the pupil (due to the tentorial herniation compressing the midbrain);
• interference with the vital functions of respiration and circulation (due to the compression of the medulla oblongata).

The dangerous downward movement at tentorial and foramen magnum levels will be encouraged by reducing the CSF pressure below the foramen magnum by lumbar puncture. Performance of a lumbar puncture may be *lethal* in these circumstances.

A mass lesion situated in the midline (Fig. 7.2b) does not have to be very large to cause obstruction to the downward flow of CSF through the ventricular system. Under such circumstances, the ventricles above the site of obstruction dilate, and both cerebral hemispheres become too large for their compartments. Bilateral tentorial herniation and coning are likely to occur with the same dangerous clinical consequences. Again, lumbar puncture may be lethal.

In the presence of a unilateral posterior fossa mass lesion, there is movement of the midline posterior fossa structures to one side. This may compress the 4th ventricle sufficiently to block the downward flow of CSF, resulting in ventricular dilatation above the site of obstruction. There will be downward movement and compression at the level of the foramen magnum. At the tentorium cerebelli, there may be

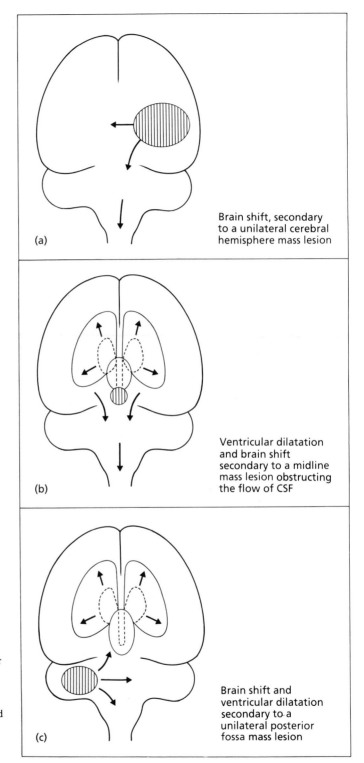

Brain shift, secondary
to a unilateral cerebral
hemisphere mass lesion

(a)

Ventricular dilatation
and brain shift
secondary to a midline
mass lesion obstructing
the flow of CSF

(b)

Brain shift and
ventricular dilatation
secondary to a
unilateral posterior
fossa mass lesion

(c)

Fig. 7.2. (a) Diagram to show the
brain shift secondary to a unilateral
cerebral hemisphere mass lesion.
(b) Diagram to show the ventricular
dilatation and brain shift
secondary to a midline mass lesion
obstructing the flow of CSF. (c)
Diagram to show the brain shift and
ventricular dilatation secondary
to a unilateral posterior fossa mass
lesion.

upward movement and compression of the midbrain or, if the supratentorial ventricular dilatation becomes very marked, there may be downward herniation bilaterally. Depression of conscious level, dilated pupils, impaired vital functions may all result from such a lesion. Again, lumbar puncture may completely decompensate a partially compensated situation with dire consequences.

Regarding the safety or otherwise of lumbar puncture in the presence of raised intracranial pressure, it is important to understand the sinister significance of the presence of a mass lesion. Where headache and papilloedema are due to a general elevation of intracranial pressure without any mass lesion, e.g. in meningitis and uncomplicated subarachnoid haemorrhage, reduction of intracranial pressure by lumbar puncture is safe and sometimes helpful in relieving symptoms. It is:
• when there is a localized mass within one of the intracranial compartments;
• when the volume of brain tissue plus mass is too large for the compartment;
• when there is shift of brain tissue out of the compartment as described above;
this is the situation which may:
• advance to serious tentorial herniation and coning;
• be accelerated to a life-threatening state by lumbar puncture.

This chapter is concerned with neoplastic intracranial mass lesions, but cerebral abscesses and intracranial haematomas behave in the same way from the point of view of compartments, shifts, herniation and coning.

We have seen that a mass lesion in one compartment of the brain can induce shift and compression in parts of the brain remote from the primary lesion. Brain tumours that are causing raised intracranial pressure are known to produce *false localizing signs*, which are no more than clinical evidence of these secondary movements of brain tissue:
• the descent of the brainstem may stretch the 6th cranial nerve to produce a non-localizing lateral rectus palsy;
• the shift away from a cerebral hemisphere mass (Fig. 7.2a) may compress the contralateral cerebral peduncle against the hard unyielding edge of the tentorial hiatus, giving rise to pyramidal signs in the limbs ipsilateral to the mass lesion;
• the ventricular dilatation above midline CSF obstructive lesions (Fig. 7.2b), or above posterior fossa lesions (Fig. 7.2c), may produce:
    — intellectual and behavioural changes suggestive of primary frontal pathology;

— an interference with vertical eye movements (which are programmed in the upper midbrain) because of the dilatation of the posterior part of the 3rd ventricle and aqueduct;
• the impairment of conscious level, pupillary dilatation and depression of vital functions, mentioned already in this chapter, are the most pressing false localizing signs and demand immediate action by doctors in charge of the case.

Clinical features

Raised intracranial pressure

We have considered in some depth one major set of symptoms and signs created by brain tumours, that is those due to raised intracranial pressure.
• Symptoms:
depression of conscious level;
headache;
vomiting.
• Signs:
depression of conscious level;
papilloedema;
false localizing signs;
signs of tentorial herniation and coning.
Only two further clinical points need to be made about these features.
1 The headaches of raised intracranial pressure tend not to be extremely severe, they do keep on troubling the patient, they are usually generalized throughout the head, and they tend to be worse in the mornings when the patient wakes. They sometimes wake the patient earlier than his normal waking time. They may be made worse by coughing, straining and bending.
2 Perfusion of the retina and optic disc may become critical in the presence of raised intracerebral pressure and papilloedema. The patient may report transient blurring or loss of vision. Such visual obscurations should stimulate urgent investigation and treatment.

Local effects

1 An *evolving focal neurological deficit*, depending on the site of the lesion. Figures 7.3 and 7.4 depict the principal neurological deficits produced by tumours situated in various parts of the brain. Tumours near the midline (Fig. 7.4) and in the posterior fossa may produce marked features of raised intracranial pressure before there are many localizing signs.

2 *Epilepsy*, in the case of supratentorial tumours. Focal epilepsy, focal epileptic activity progressing to grand mal, grand mal epilepsy with a transient localizing aura, grand mal epilepsy with post-ictal focal neurological signs, and grand mal epilepsy without any apparent focal features may all indicate the presence of a tumour in the cerebrum. (Epilepsy is not a feature of posterior fossa tumours.)

Epilepsy is not commonly caused by tumours, and considerably less than 50% of cerebral tumours produce epilepsy, but the occurrence of epilepsy should prompt the possibility of a brain tumour in the doctor's mind. This is especially true:

• if there are focal neurological signs;

• if the patient is over 20 years and has no family history of epilepsy, no previous history of epilepsy in early life, and no history of any condition (e.g. head injury, meningitis) earlier in life which might have created an epileptogenic lesion.

Fig. 7.3. Lateral aspect of the brain, showing the neurological deficits produced by tumours at various sites.

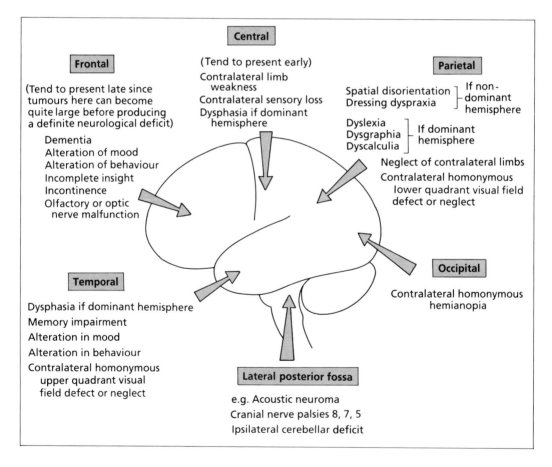

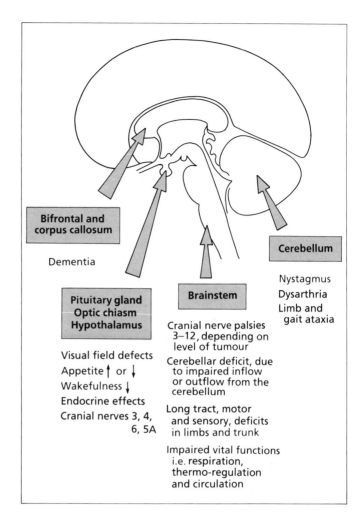

Fig. 7.4. Median section through the brain, showing the neurological deficits produced by tumours at various sites.

The diagram shows labels and their associated deficits:

Bifrontal and corpus callosum

Dementia

Pituitary gland Optic chiasm Hypothalamus

Visual field defects
Appetite ↑ or ↓
Wakefulness ↓
Endocrine effects
Cranial nerves 3, 4, 6, 5A

Brainstem

Cranial nerve palsies 3–12, depending on level of tumour

Cerebellar deficit, due to impaired inflow or outflow from the cerebellum

Long tract, motor and sensory, deficits in limbs and trunk

Impaired vital functions i.e. respiration, thermo-regulation and circulation

Cerebellum

Nystagmus
Dysarthria
Limb and gait ataxia

Common brain tumours

Benign

- Grade 1–2 gliomas
- Meningioma
- Pituitary adenoma
- Acoustic neuroma

Malignant

Primary
- Grade 3–4 gliomas
Secondary
- Metastatic carcinoma

Gliomas are seen to appear in both the benign and malignant groups of tumours. Each of the three glial cells,

85   *Brain tumour*

astrocytes, oligodendrocytes and microglia, may undergo neoplastic change. Astrocytomas are more common than oligodendrogliomas, and microgliomas are rare. Gliomas are classified histologically from grade 1 (benign) to grade 4 (the highly malignant glioblastoma multiforme). Benign gliomas are, unfortunately, much less common than malignant ones.

Meningiomas are nearly always benign. They may arise from any part of the meninges, over the surface of the brain, from the falx, or from the tentorium. There is a plane of cleavage between tumour and brain tissue which makes total removal a definite possibility, so long as the tumour is reasonably accessible and unattached to dural venous sinuses, e.g. the sagittal sinus.

Pituitary adenomas produce two principal sets of symptoms: space-occupying effects and endocrine disturbance. When the pituitary gland enlarges in the pituitary fossa, it most commonly expands upwards (suprasellar extension) to compress optic nerves/chiasm/tracts. The classical bitemporal hemianopia resulting from chiasmal compression occurs when the optic chiasm is right above a pituitary extension which is directly upwards. The exact position of the optic chiasm, and the direction of pituitary expansion, do, however, vary from one case to another, so monocular blindness due to optic nerve compression and homonymous hemianopia from optic tract compression are not uncommon in patients with pituitary adenomas. Lateral expansion of pitiutary adenomas may compress structures on the lateral wall of the cavernous sinus (cranial nerves 3, 4, 5a and 6), producing double vision and forehead numbness. Forward and downward expansion of the adenoma results in enormous expansion of the pitiutary fossa and occasional erosion through bone into the sphenoidal air sinus.

The endocrinological disturbances that accompany the development of a pituitary adenoma are *positive* if the tumour cells are secretory (prolactin, growth hormone, etc.), and *negative* if the tumour is preventing normal secretion by the rest of the pituitary gland (varying degrees of panhypopituitarism).

Acoustic neuromas are benign tumours of the Schwann cells along the course of the acoustic nerve, between the cerebellopontine angle and the internal auditory meatus in the petrous temporal bone. First and foremost, they produce progressive unilateral nerve deafness, but by the time of recognition there may well be associated 5th and 7th nerve dysfunction, unilateral cerebellar signs and evidence of raised intracranial pressure. Early diagnosis is highly desirable since a small tumour is much safer to remove from the posterior fossa than a large one which has become associated with brainstem displacement and raised intracranial pressure.

The *common malignant tumours* in the brain are either *gliomas* or *metastases*, in particular malignant astrocytomas and metastatic carcinoma. Together these constitute well over 60% of all brain tumours. The history is usually short, of raised intracranial pressure, epilepsy or neurological deficit. Not uncommonly, all three groups of symptoms are present by the time of diagnosis. It is not uncommon for a primary carcinoma elsewhere in the body to present with metastatic disease in the brain. If the metastases are multiple, the differentiation from malignant glioma is not difficult, but solitary cerebral metastases are quite commonly seen in practice.

Rarer brain tumours

Benign

- Optic glioma
- Craniopharyngioma
- Colloid cyst and choroid plexus papilloma
- Haemangioblastoma
- Cerebellar cystic astrocytoma
- Neuroma on a cranial nerve other than 8

Malignant

Primary
- Ependymoma
- Medulloblastoma

Secondary
- Metastatic melanoma
- Lymphoma
- Malignant meningeal infiltration
            (*NB* These lists are not comprehensive.)

Optic glioma and *craniopharyngioma* usually present with visual deficits. There may be associated hypothalamic or pituitary malfunction.

Colloid cysts and *papillomas arising from the choroid plexus* are intraventricular tumours capable of producing chronic, intermittent or acute blockage to CSF pathways.

Haemangioblastoma is a benign cystic tumour which occurs in the cerebellum most frequently. It is a tumour found in adult patients.

Cerebellar cystic astrocytoma is a posterior fossa tumour seen in childhood with excellent prognosis; *ependymoma* and *medulloblastoma* are much more sinister posterior fossa tumours in children.

The trigeminal nerve is the only other cranial nerve to develop a *neuroma*.

Metastatic melanoma in the brain carries the same appalling prognosis as it does elsewhere in the body.

Cerebral lymphoma is seen more commonly in immunosuppressed patients, and is therefore increasing in frequency.

Carcinoma, leukaemia and lymphoma may sometimes infiltrate the meninges along the spinal canal and around the brain, to produce a chronic progressive *malignant meningitis*, rather than forming a solid deposit of malignant tissue. This uncommon disorder presents with multiple cranial or spinal nerve lesions, sometimes associated with raised intracranial pressure.

Differential diagnosis

The common presenting symptoms of brain tumours are:
- raised intracranial pressure;
- epilepsy;
- a progressive focal neurological deficit.

Clearly, other mass lesions within the head may produce *all three features*. There may be difficulty in differentiating a malignant tumour from an intracerebral abscess when the history is a short one, and from subdural haematoma or intracranial granuloma (e.g. sarcoid) when the history is a little longer.

Raised intracranial pressure

Other causes of raised intracranial pressure include arterial hypertension, chronic meningitis and benign intracranial hypertension (which is a curious elevation of intracranial pressure in the absence of any obvious cause, chiefly found in young overweight females).

Epilepsy and focal epilepsy

Epilepsy and focal epilepsy are more usually caused by epileptogenic scars from previous intracranial disease, e.g. trauma, meningitis, etc.

Progressive focal neurological deficit

The principal alternative cause of a progressive focal neurological deficit is an ischaemic stroke, which, instead of developing with characteristic abruptness, comes on in a stuttering way. It is sometimes difficult, therefore, to be sure whether a patient is suffering from internal carotid atheromatous disease or a malignant neoplasm in the cerebral hemisphere. Occasionally, a sudden bleed can occur in a malignant brain tumour, so that the case presents as a patient with a primary intracerebral haemorrhage.

Investigation

If the clinical presentation suggests the likelihood of a brain tumour, *admission to hospital* for further investigation is indicated in most cases. Admission to a neurological or neurosurgical unit under these circumstances is likely to be extremely stressful to the patient and relatives. Reassurance, sympathy, and encouragement together with adequate explanation are required. Clearly, admission to hospital will not be as immediate in patients presenting with epilepsy, as in the case of a patient showing a progressing neurological deficit and clear evidence of raised intracranial pressure.

Computerized tomography scanning

CT scanning, before and after injection of intravascular contrast material, is the main diagnostic investigation. This technique will demonstrate the presence of the vast majority of brain tumours, and indicate the extent of any shift and ventricular dilatation that may have been caused. How much cerebral oedema has been generated by the presence of the neoplasm will also be apparent. CT scanning may require the support of:
• plain radiographs of the skull (looking for evidence of raised intracranial pressure or bony erosion);
• radiological and other imaging techniques elsewhere in the body if metastatic disease seems likely;
• carotid or vertebral angiography if the neurosurgical team needs this information prior to surgery;
• haematological and biochemical investigation if cerebral abscess, granuloma, metastatic disease or pituitary pathology are under consideration.

Magnetic resonance scanning

Magnetic resonance scanning may occasionally detect or give better definition of an intracranial tumour than can be achieved by CT scanning. This is particularly true of tumours in or near the base of the skull.

(*NB* Lumbar puncture is contra-indicated in suspected cases of cerebral tumour.)

89 *Brain tumour*

Management

If the patient shows marked features of raised intracranial pressure and CT scanning displays considerable cerebral oedema, dexamethasone may be used with considerable benefit. The patient will be relieved of unpleasant, and sometimes dangerous, symptoms and signs, and the intracranial state made much safer if neurosurgical intervention is to be undertaken.

Surgical management

What can the neurosurgeon do for the common types of brain tumour?

Complete removal

Meningiomas, pituitary tumours not susceptible to medical treatment, acoustic neuromas and some solitary metastases in accessible regions of the brain can all be removed completely. Sometimes, the neurosurgical operation required is long and difficult if the benign tumour is relatively inaccessible.

Partial removal

Gliomas in the frontal, occipital and temporal poles may be removed by fairly radical de-bulking operations. Sometimes, benign tumours cannot be removed in their entirety because of tumour position or patient frailty.

Biopsy

If at all possible, the histological nature of any mass lesion in the brain should be established. What looks like a glioma or metastasis from the clinical and CT points of view occasionally turns out to be an abscess, a benign tumour or granuloma. If the mass lesion is not in a part of the brain where partial removal can be attempted, biopsy by means of a needle through a burrhole usually establishes the histological diagnosis. The accuracy and safety of this procedure may be increased by use of stereotactic surgical techniques. Histological confirmation may not be mandatory where there is strong collateral evidence of metastatic disease.

Histological confirmation may be postponed in patients presenting with epilepsy only, in whom a rather small mass lesion in an inaccessible part of the brain is revealed by CT scan. Sequential CT scanning, initially at short intervals, may be the most reasonable management plan in such patients.

Shunting

Inaccessible midline tumours causing ventricular dilatation may be treated successfully by insertion of a ventriculo-atrial or ventriculo-peritoneal shunt. This allows the intracranial pressure to return to normal. Raised intracranial pressure may have been the only problem produced by some such tumours.

Additional forms of treatment

Radiotherapy

Middle-grade gliomas, metastases, and pituitary adenomas are the common intracranial tumours which are radiosensitive. The posterior fossa malignant tumours of childhood and lymphoma are also sensitive to radiotherapy. Radiotherapy commonly follows partial removal or biopsy of such lesions, and continues over a few weeks whilst the pre-operative dose of dexamethasone is being gradually reduced.

Chemotherapy

No really effective antimitotic agents have been found yet for brain tumours, with the possible exception of lymphoma.

Anticonvulsants

Control of epilepsy may be an important part of the management of a patient with a supratentorial brain tumour.

Dexamethasone

Taken in large and constant dosage, dexamethasone may be the most humane treatment of patients with highly malignant gliomas or metastatic disease. Used in this way, dexamethasone often allows significant symptomatic relief so that the patient can return home and enjoy a short period of dignified existence before the tumour once more shows its presence. At this point, dexamethasone can be withdrawn and opiates used as required.

Prognosis

The fact that the majority of brain tumours are either malignant gliomas or metastases, which obviously carry a very poor prognosis, hangs like a cloud over the outlook for patients with the common brain tumours.

91   *Brain tumour*

Table 7.1

Grade	Tumour	Treatment	Outcome
Benign	Grade 1–2 gliomas Meningioma Pituitary adenoma Acoustic neuroma	Complete removal, plus radiotherapy for pituitary adenoma, *or*	'Cure', but often with some residual neurological deficit
		Incomplete removal, plus radiotherapy for pituitary adenoma	Survival for many years, often with some residual neurological deficit. Eventual reappearance of tumour which may be difficult to treat on the second occasion
Malignant	Grade 3–4 gliomas Metastatic carcinoma	Complete removal, incomplete removal, biopsy, plus or minus radiotherapy, dexamethasone	Only a small percentage of 2-year survivors, and considerable morbidity during the survival period

Table 7.1 summarizes the outlook for patients with the common brain tumours. It can be seen that such pessimism is justified for malignant brain tumours, but not for the less common benign neoplasms.

Chapter 8

Head injury

The cause

Road traffic accidents involving car drivers, car passengers, motor-cycle drivers and pillion-seat riders, cyclists, pedestrians and runners constitute the single greatest cause of head injury in Western society. Compulsory speed limits, car seat-belts and motor-cycle helmets, stricter control over driving after drinking alcohol, and clothing to make cyclists and runners more visible have all proved helpful in preventing road accidents, yet road accidents are still responsible for more head injuries than any other source.

Accidents at work account for a significant number of head injuries, despite the greater use of protective headgear. Sport, especially horse-riding, constitutes a further source of head injury. Accidents around the home account for an unfortunate number of head injuries, especially in young children who are unable to take proper precautions with open windows, ladders, stairs and bunk-beds. Child abuse has to be remembered as a possible cause of head injury to ensure that such trauma is prevented from happening again.

It is a sad fact that head injury, trivial and severe, affects young people in significant numbers. Approximately 50% of patients admitted to hospital on account of head injury in the United Kingdom are under the age of 20 years. This no doubt indicates the susceptibility of young children to accidents at home, the involvement of young people in sport, the recklessness of youth when driving cars and motor-cycles, and the irresponsibility of young people in their consumption of alcohol.

The effect in pathological terms

The brain is an organ of relatively soft consistency contained in a rigid, compartmentalized, unyielding box which has a rough and irregular bottom. Sudden acceleration, deceleration or rotation certainly allow movement of the brain within the skull. If sudden and massive enough, such

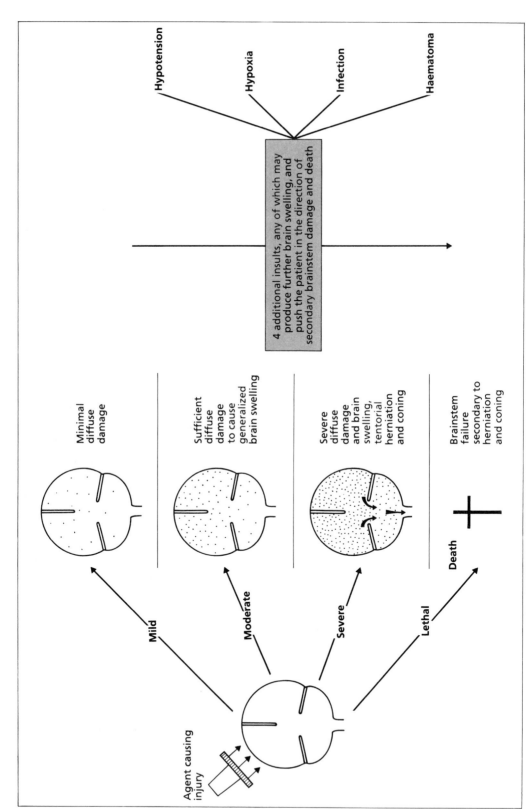

Fig. 8.1. A summary of the pathological effects that may occur as a consequence of head injury.

movement will cause tearing of nerve fibres and petechial haemorrhages within the white matter, and contusions and lacerations of the cortex especially over the base of the brain.

If the trauma has been severe, the diffuse damage to the brain described above may cause generalized brain swelling, just like the swelling that occurs with injury to any other organ. The fact that the brain is contained within a rigid box is, however, different to other organs of the body. Diffuse brain swelling may result in the brain becoming too large in volume for the space allocated to it. As discussed at the beginning of Chapter 7, this may lead to tentorial herniation, midbrain compression, impaction of the lower medulla and cerebellar hemispheres in the foramen magnum, secondary brainstem pathology, and death (see Fig. 8.1).

In the circumstances of head injury, the diffusely damaged brain is extremely vulnerable to four other insults, all of which produce further brain swelling (see Fig. 8.1). By causing further swelling, each of the four insults listed below tend to encourage the downward cascade towards brainstem failure and death:

1 arterial hypotension — from blood loss at the time of injury, possibly from the scalp but more probably from an associated injury elsewhere in the body. Hypotension will lead to ischaemic cerebral oedema;

2 arterial hypoxia — because of airway obstruction or associated chest injury. Hypoxia will cause hypoxic cerebral oedema;

3 infection — head injuries in which skull fracture has occurred may allow organisms to enter the skull via an open wound, or from the ear or nose. Infection causes inflammatory oedema;

4 intracranial haematoma — the force of injury may have torn a blood vessel inside the skull (either in the brain substance or in the meninges) so that a haematoma forms. This causes further compression of the brain by taking up volume within the rigid skull.

The effect in clinical terms

The clinical instrument that is used to monitor the effects of head injury on patients requiring admission to hospital is the neurological observation chart created by competent, trained nursing staff.

This chart includes the patient's responsiveness using the Glasgow Coma Scale, recording the patient's best eye, verbal and motor responses, together with his vital signs of

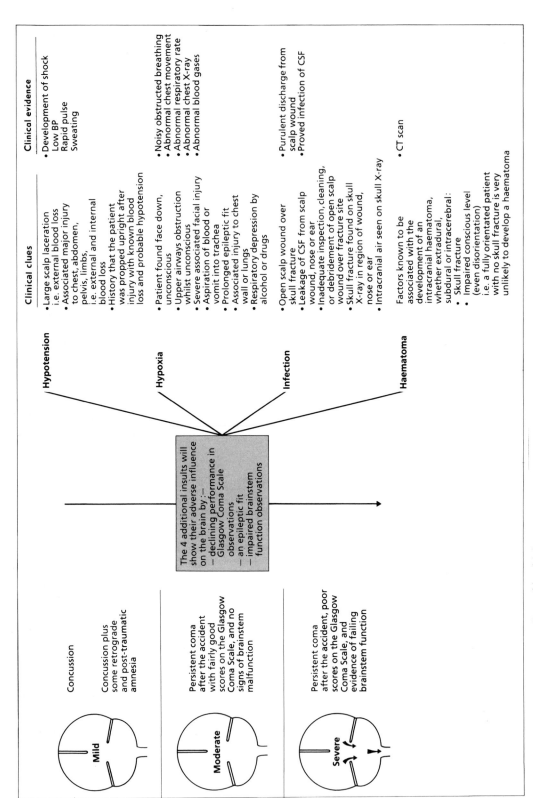

		Clinical clues	Clinical evidence
Mild	Concussion Concussion plus some retrograde and post-traumatic amnesia		
Moderate	Persistent coma after the accident with fairly good scores on the Glasgow Coma Scale, and no signs of brainstem malfunction		
Severe	Persistent coma after the accident, poor scores on the Glasgow Coma Scale, and evidence of failing brainstem function		

The 4 additional insults will show their adverse influence on the brain by:—
— declining performance in Glasgow Coma Scale observations
— an epileptic fit
— impaired brainstem function observations

Hypotension
- Large scalp laceration i.e. external blood loss
- Associated major injury to chest, abdomen, pelvis, limbs, i.e. external and internal blood loss
- History that the patient was propped upright after injury with known blood loss and probable hypotension

Clinical evidence:
- Development of shock Low BP Rapid pulse Sweating

Hypoxia
- Patient found face down, unconscious
- Upper airways obstruction whilst unconscious
- Severe associated facial injury
- Aspiration of blood or vomit into trachea
- Prolonged epileptic fit
- Associated injury to chest wall or lungs
- Respiratory depression by alcohol or drugs

Clinical evidence:
- Noisy obstructed breathing
- Abnormal chest movement
- Abnormal respiratory rate
- Abnormal chest X-ray
- Abnormal blood gases

Infection
- Open scalp wound over skull fracture
- Leakage of CSF from scalp wound, nose or ear
- Inadequate inspection, cleaning, or debridement of open scalp wound over fracture site
- Skull fracture found on skull X-ray in region of wound, nose or ear
- Intracranial air seen on skull X-ray

Clinical evidence:
- Purulent discharge from scalp wound
- Proved infection of CSF

Haematoma
- Factors known to be associated with the development of an intracranial haematoma, whether extradural, subdural or intracerebral:
  - Skull fracture
  - Impaired conscious level (even disorientation)
  i.e. a fully orientated patient with no skull fracture is very unlikely to develop a haematoma

Clinical evidence:
- CT scan

Fig. 8.2. A summary of the clinical effects of head injury.

pupil size and reactivity, blood pressure, pulse, respiratory rate and temperature. The observations are made at intervals appropriate to the patient's clinical condition — every 15 minutes in critically ill patients.

The Glasgow Coma Scale requires the observer to record the patient's:

- best eye-opening response:
  spontaneous;
  to speech;
  to pain;
  none;
- best verbal response:
  orientated;
  confused conversation;
  short inappropriate exclamations;
  incomprehensible moans and groans;
  none;
- best motor response (usually recorded in the best arm):
  obeys verbal commands;
  localizes painful stimulus;
  limb flexion in response to pain;
  limb extension in response to pain;
  none.

A diagram showing the use of the Glasgow Coma Scale (Fig. 1.3) appears in Chapter 1 (page 10). Changes in these chart observations are used to signal changes in the patient's brain condition with great sensitivity.

The vital signs of pupil size and reactivity, blood pressure, pulse, respiratory rate, and temperature are, essentially, indicators of brainstem function.

Figure 8.2 shows the clinical states that accompany mild, moderate and severe degrees of diffuse cerebral damage after head injury. The adverse influence of hypotension, hypoxia, infection and intracranial haematoma will become apparent in the patient's chart observations, possibly accompanied by an epileptic fit. The appearance of abnormal brainstem signs indicates that the additional insult is adversely affecting the brain very seriously.

Figure 8.2 also shows the clinical clues, and definite signs, that confirm the presence of one or more of the four additional insults. Ideally, the clues should make the doctor so alert to the possibility of the insult becoming operational that the problem is rectified before the patient starts to decline significantly in his Glasgow Coma Scale observations, and certainly before evidence of impaired brainstem function appears.

Management

Patients with head injury require management in three situations: the hospital accident department (or general practitioner's surgery), the surgical ward experienced in the care of head injuries, and the neurosurgical unit (see Fig. 8.3).

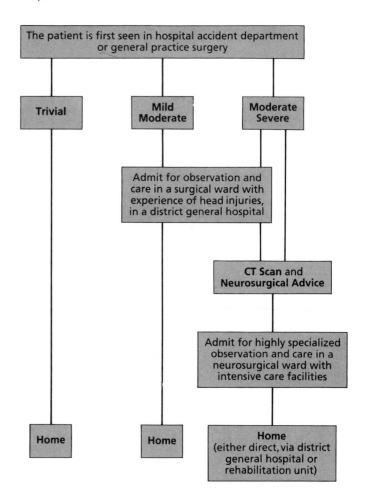

Fig. 8.3. A logistic plan showing the management of patients with head injury.

1 Hospital accident department or general practice surgery

- Has there been loss of consciousness or amnesia at any time?
- Are there any neurological symptoms or signs?
- Is there blood or CSF leaking from the ear or nose?
- Is there a suspicion of penetrating injury?
- Is there scalp bruising or swelling?

If the answer to *all* of the above questions is **no**, the patient has a *trivial head injury* and can be allowed home in the

company of a responsible adult who:
- will check the patient at intervals for drowsiness, confusion, or severe headache;
- knows not to give the patient anything other than simple analgesics;
- is able to bring the patient back to the hospital urgently if necessary.

If the answer to *any* of the above questions is **yes**, the patient has a *mild, moderate, or severe head injury.*
1 Arrange a skull X-ray.
2 Consider admission.

Admit the patient to hospital if the answer to any of the following questions is **yes**.
- Is there confusion, or any other evidence of impaired consciousness, at the time of examination in the accident room or surgery?
- Is there a skull fracture?
- Is there blood or CSF leaking from the ear or nose?
- Is there evidence of a penetrating injury?
- Are any neurological symptoms or signs present?
- Are there factors present which make assessment of the patient uncertain? (e.g. young child, alcohol, epilepsy)
- Does the patient lack a responsible adult who can observe him and return him to hospital urgently if necessary?

2 Surgical ward of district general hospital

- Establish regular competent *neurological observations* at intervals appropriate to the patient's condition (half-hourly, hourly, 2-hourly, 4-hourly).
- Remember the head injury may be *non-accidental.* If there is any uncertainty about the mechanism of head injury, remember that the patient may have injured his head as a consequence of:
  stroke;
  cerebral haemorrhage;
  epilepsy;
  cardiac dysrhythmia;
  alcoholic intoxication;
  non-accidental injury.
- Remember that there are *pharmacological dangers.* If the patient smells of alcohol, the doctor may recognize that this could be a contributory factor towards the patient's depressed state of consciousness, but he will be unwise to attribute the whole clinical picture to alcohol if a head injury is present, especially if a skull fracture is present.

99   *Head injury*

Do not complicate the state of consciousness, or the assessment of it, by:
  — the use of strong, CNS depressant, analgesics;
  — the overuse of intravenous CNS depressant drugs to control an individual epileptic fit;
  — permitting any procedures requiring general anaesthesia, which can possibly wait for two or three days;
  — the use of mydriatic drugs to look at the fundi.
• Anticipate, prevent, detect early, and treat energetically any of the *four serious insults* which may further damage the brain and cause further brain swelling.

1 *Hypotension:* Recognize the possibility of external and internal blood loss from the scalp or from an associated injury elsewhere in the body. Attend to shock swiftly by fluid or blood replacement, elevation of the foot of the bed, intravenous dopamine, etc.

2 *Hypoxia:* Attend to upper airway and recognize any chest wall or lung injury. Remember the possibility of aspiration and respiratory depression by alcohol or drugs. Chest X-ray and arterial blood gas estimation are not expensive investigations!

3 *Infection:* Pay extreme care to the correct treatment of an open wound over a skull fracture. Look for CSF leakage at such a wound and from the nose or ear (especially if there is a fracture in the floor of the anterior cranial fossa or petrous temporal bone). Look for intracranial air on the patient's skull X-ray. Look for any evidence of scalp wound infection.

4 *Haematoma:* Remember that the presence of a skull fracture elevates the risk of an intracerebral haematoma very significantly, especially if associated with any impairment of conscious level. These patients are the patients who may need to be examined by CT scan, unless there are special reasons, e.g. significant injuries to other parts of the body, making it difficult to move the patient.

3 Accident department or surgical ward

A *CT scan* should be performed and *neurosurgical advice* should be sought under the following circumstances:
• the patient has a skull fracture, and shows confusion or other evidence of a depressed conscious level;
• the patient has a skull fracture, and suffers one or more epileptic fits;
• the patient has a skull fracture, and has any other neurological symptoms or signs;
• the patient's coma persists after initial resuscitation, even though there may be no skull fracture;

- a deterioration in conscious level occurs, evidenced by falling scores on the Glasgow Coma Scale;
- confusion or other neurological disturbance persists for more than 8 hours, even though there may be no skull fracture;
- there is a depressed fracture of the skull vault;
- there is a suspected or proved fracture of the skull base, (CSF rhinorrhoea or otorrhoea, bilateral orbital haematoma, mastoid haematoma);
- there is evidence of penetrating or missile type of injury.

4 Neurosurgical unit

- *Neurological observations* will be performed by extremely skilled nursing staff at short intervals, e.g. every 15 minutes.
- The same care over the use of any *drugs* with CNS depressant effects and general anaesthetics will be taken as mentioned on page 100.
- The same anticipation and early energetic treatment of the *four main insults* to the damaged brain will occur, as mentioned on page 100, including CT scan detection of brain swelling and intracranial haematoma.
- Agents to *reduce brain swelling* will be used, if brain swelling endangers the patient. Cerebral oedema is reduced by intermittent intravenous injections of mannitol, or by elective hyperventilation (dexamethasone is not good at reducing the oedema which accompanies cerebral damage caused by head injury). Haematoma evacuation may be necessary, especially extradural haematoma.
- The *routine care of the unconscious patient,* described in detail in Chapter 1 (page 13), will be established.

After-care

In all but the most trivial head injuries, the patient will benefit from some after-care. This may not amount to more than simple explanation and reassurance regarding a period of amnesia, headaches, uncertainty about a skull fracture, timing of return to work, etc. Without the opportunity to discuss such matters, unnecessary apprehensions may persist in the mind of the patient and his family.

At the other end of the scale, somebody recovering from a major head injury (often associated with other injuries) may need a great deal of further medical and paramedical care for months after the head injury. This may mean a considerable period in hospital or in a rehabilitation unit whilst recovery from the intellectual, psychological, neurological and orthopaedic deficits gradually occurs.

The consequences

How severe a head injury was it, Doctor?

The answer to this question must take note of several factors, all of which should be remembered in formulating a reply.

- Initial features:
  level of consciousness;
  skull fracture;
  focal neurological signs.
- Secondary features:
  epilepsy;
  intracranial haematoma;
  meningitis.
- Duration:
  of coma;
  of post-traumatic amnesia;
  of stay in hospital.
- Persisting deficits:
  intellectual;
  psychological;
  focal neurological.

With regard to the duration of coma and post-traumatic amnesia, confusion may arise. The duration of post-traumatic amnesia refers to the period after the accident until the time that the patient regains ongoing memory. The patient often describes the latter as the time he woke up after the accident. He means the time he recovered his memory, not the time he recovered consciousness. The time *he* says he woke up is often long after the time that observers have noted return of consciousness (eyes open and paying attention, speaking and using his limbs purposefully).

The duration of hospital stay must also be clarified. If there was associated (orthopaedic) injury, the patient may have been hospitalized long after the time for discharge purely on head injury grounds.

Post-concussion syndrome

This usually follows minor concussive head injury with post-traumatic amnesic periods lasting a few minutes, rather than major head injury. It consists of a remarkably stereotyped set of symptoms, unaccompanied by abnormal neurological signs:

- headache;
- dizziness;
- impaired concentration;
- impaired memory;
- fatigue;
- anxiety;
- depression;
- irritability;
- indecisiveness;
- impaired self-confidence;
- lack of drive;
- impaired libido

'I can't get going after that accident . . . . headaches every day, and nothing seems to be working properly'

Controversy exists as to the cause of the post-concussion syndrome. On the one hand, it is accepted that concussive head injury can produce diffuse minor brain damage. (If repeated, this may accumulate to the punch-drunk state, known as post-traumatic encephalopathy, seen in some boxers towards the end of their careers.) On the other hand, the syndrome can be seen in some patients suffering head injuries at work, where the evidence of concussion or amnesia is very minimal and where litigation and financial compensation are paramount.

The syndrome can be very disabling for months, even years, after a minor head injury. Despite our lack of understanding of its precise nature, the syndrome has to be recognized as a definite entity responsible for considerable morbidity after head injury in some patients.

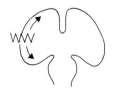

Post-traumatic epilepsy

Patients surviving head injury may have developed an epileptogenic scar in the brain, which may subsequently give rise to focal or generalized epileptic attacks. Post-traumatic epilepsy shows its presence within a year of the accident in about 50% of patients who are going to develop this late complication of their head injury. In the rest, it may not occur for several years.

There are certain features of the head injury which make post-traumatic epilepsy more likely:
• post-traumatic amnesia lasting more than 24 hours;
• focal neurological signs during the week after the head injury;
• epilepsy during the week after the head injury;
• depressed skull fracture;
• dural tear;
• intracranial haematoma.
These risk factors enable fairly accurate prediction of the risk of epilepsy in a patient after head injury, and are valuable when advising patients about prophylactic anticonvulsants and driving.

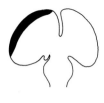

Chronic subdural haematoma

In elderly patients who have suffered trivial head injury, sometimes so trivial that it is not clearly remembered, blood may start to collect in the subdural space. This is not sudden, severe arterial bleeding, but a process that evolves over several weeks, a gradual accumulation and liquefaction of blood. The blood accumulates over the convexity of the brain, with gradual elevation of intracranial pressure, shift of midline structures and eventual tentorial herniation and coning.

The clinical picture is of subacute fluctuating drowsiness and confusion, often associated with headache, in which focal neurological signs appear late. Any elderly patient presenting in this way is a candidate for a chronic subdural haematoma, with or without a history of head injury. Chronic alcoholics and patients on anticoagulants have an increased risk of chronic subdural haematoma.

Chronic subdural haematomas may occur bilaterally, and may be hard to visualize on conventional CT scans, the altered blood being isodense with brain tissue. They are treated by evacuation of the blood through burrholes, with good results.

Outcome from severe head injury

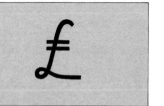

Mortality from severe head injury (coma lasting more than 6 hours) is of the order of 50%. Those who survive are likely to have deficits in some or all of the following areas, depending on which parts of the brain have been most damaged:
- intellectual function;
- mood, behaviour, personality;
- speech and communication;
- vision;
- neuromuscular function.

Most of a patient's recovery will have occurred within 6 months of the injury, though further slower improvement may occur in the next 12–18 months.

Patients displaying deficits in all areas constitute what the general public recognize as a brain-damaged person, often unable to live independently. Commonly, the patients are young at the time of their accident, and many years of life may lie ahead of them. In general, provision for such patients is inadequate in terms of chronic young sick units, where their ongoing care may be successfully managed in some sort of shared care system with the patient's relatives.

Compensation and medico-legal aspects

Because road traffic accidents and accidents at work cause a large percentage of head injuries, compensation for suffering, disability, loss of earnings, restriction in recreational pursuits, etc. is very commonly sought in the months and years after the accident. This occurs after both minor and major injuries, and it is unusual for a case to be settled before two years have elapsed after the accident.

Though this activity is entirely reasonable, it is unsettling for the patient and his family. It tends to perpetuate the accident and its effects in their minds longer than would otherwise be the case.

Chapter 9

Tremor; abnormal, involuntary, and clumsy movement

Introduction

This chapter is about a variety of disparate conditions in which some form of involuntary, clumsy or imperfect movement occurs. For simplicity, the different syndromes are described in their purest forms, though in clinical practice such patients are sometimes difficult to classify. This is either because features of their disorder are not 'classical', or because features of more than one type of disorder are found in the same patient.

It will be recalled from Chapter 5 that normal, smooth, well-coordinated movement relies upon the integrity of the primary motor pathway (upper motor neurone–lower motor neurone–neuromuscular junction–muscle), supported by perfectly normal cerebellar, basal ganglion and sensory function, especially proprioceptive sense, as shown in Fig. 9.1.

Most patients with tremors, involuntary and clumsy movement have normal strength, reflecting the fact that the primary motor pathway is intact. Their disorders involve, therefore, cerebellar, basal ganglion or sensory malfunction.

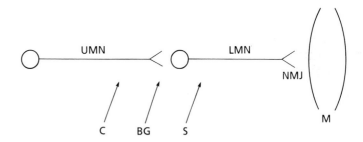

UMN = Upper motor neurone
LMN = Lower motor neurone
NMJ = Neuromuscular junction
M = Muscle
C = Cerebellum
BG = Basal ganglia
S = Sensation

Fig. 9.1. Diagram to show the basic components of the nervous system required for normal movement.

Tremor

Involuntary movements that are rhythmic or fairly rhythmic, whether of large amplitude or barely visible, are grouped under the general term tremor. A classification of the common forms of tremor is shown in Fig. 9.2.

The important differentiating feature of the tremor of Parkinson's disease is the fact that it is most evident at rest. It is reduced or eliminated by voluntary movement. The other features of Parkinson's disease, bradykinesia and cogwheel rigidity, which are nearly always present to some degree, aid accurate diagnostic categorization of patients with this form of tremor.

Patients with cerebellar lesions commonly have clumsy, uncoordinated movement of their limbs. Frequently, this lack of smooth coordination of muscle activity is most evident in the limbs on attempted accurate placement of the distal part of the limb, e.g. placing the finger on the nose, or placing the heel on the opposite knee. The incoordination is present throughout the proximal and distal muscles, leading to large-amplitude, random, non-rhythmic shaking of the limb. Such movement is unlikely to be confused with other kinds of tremor. A few patients with lesions in the superior cerebellar peduncle will show rhythmic tremor. This is usually a large-amplitude, slow rhythmic tremor, present in head, body and limbs, absent at rest, present during any movement, and made much worse by attempted accurate limb placement. It is most commonly caused by multiple sclerosis.

The other large group of action tremors are really exaggerations of normal physiological tremor. They are usually faster than parkinsonian or cerebellar tremors, absent at rest, and present through the whole range of any movement. They are most evident distally, especially in the hands.

Physiological tremor is made more evident when circulating catecholamines are increased. How and why catecholamines do this is not clearly understood; possibly they have an effect on muscle contraction time, or possibly an effect in the spinal cord. Physiological tremor, whether normal or exaggerated, does respond to beta-adrenergic blockade. Surgeons, marksmen and musicians have discovered this, and commonly reduce their physiological tremor for an important occasion by taking propranolol. Several of the exaggerated physiological tremors, identified in the right-

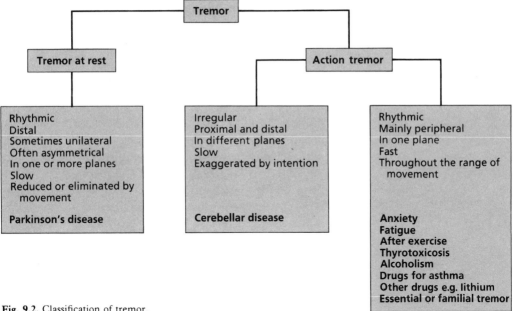

```
                          ┌─────────┐
                          │ Tremor  │
                          └─────────┘
          ┌──────────────────┴──────────────────┐
   ┌───────────────┐                    ┌───────────────┐
   │ Tremor at rest│                    │ Action tremor │
   └───────────────┘                    └───────────────┘
                                    ┌──────────┴──────────┐
```

Rhythmic	Irregular	Rhythmic
Distal	Proximal and distal	Mainly peripheral
Sometimes unilateral	In different planes	In one plane
Often asymmetrical	Slow	Fast
In one or more planes	Exaggerated by intention	Throughout the range of
Slow		movement
Reduced or eliminated by		
movement		
Parkinson's disease	**Cerebellar disease**	**Anxiety**
		Fatigue
		After exercise
		Thyrotoxicosis
		Alcoholism
		Drugs for asthma
		Other drugs e.g. lithium
		Essential or familial tremor

Fig. 9.2. Classification of tremor.

hand column of Fig. 9.2, are also helped by beta-blockers, e.g. patients with anxiety or thyrotoxicosis, and patients with benign essential or familial tremor. The sympathomimetic drugs used in patients with asthma not infrequently cause tremor.

A small dose of alcohol also settles an exaggerated physiological tremor. Some people 'steady their nerves' with a small drink before an important occasion. Alcoholics may settle their morning tremor with a drink, and some patients with benign essential or familial tremor find that their hands shake less when reaching for the second glass of sherry.

Parkinson's disease

After cerebrovascular disease, Parkinson's disease and multiple sclerosis are the two most common neurological disorders producing physical disability in the UK. Parkinson's disease is increasing in incidence in line with increased longevity. It is also rising in prevalence as effective treatment for the condition continues to improve.

Idiopathic Parkinson's disease is the result of one particular pattern of loss of nerve cells from the central nervous system. Initially, and for years, this may be confined to the neurones of the substantia nigra, though later in the illness neuronal loss may occur from other basal ganglion and brainstem nuclei. The cause of this neuronal degeneration is not known, and treatment of the condition does not alter the continued loss of further nerve cells.

The loss of cells from the central nervous system in Parkinson's disease occurs at a variable rate and to a variable extent. Thus, some patients become rapidly disabled within a few years, whilst others have a mild, faintly progressive disorder for many years requiring little or no treatment. The majority of cases come between these two extremes, suffering a condition which slowly becomes more and more intrusive over a period of about 10 years. Most patients present after the age of 50 years. Without treatment, the average time from diagnosis to death is 9 years. The quality of life and life expectancy for patients have both increased over the last 15 years as a consequence of L-dopa therapy.

The neurones of the substantia nigra project to the corpus striatum via the nigro-striatal pathway. This is dopaminergic. The consequence of loss of neurones in the substantia nigra is dopamine deficiency in the corpus striatum. The corpus striatum is left in a state of inadequate dopaminergic stimulation, yet remains more normally stimulated by other neurotransmitters, most notably acetylcholine. The influences of dopamine and acetylcholine in the corpus striatum appear to be opposite to each other. When the corpus striatum is very deficient in dopamine stimulation (therefore relatively overstimulated by cholinergic pathways), the parkinsonian syndrome ensues (see Fig. 9.3). Nigro-striatal failure may be unilateral, asymmetrical or symmetrical.

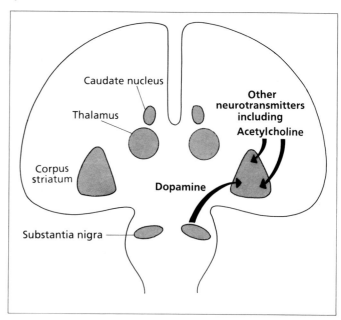

Fig. 9.3. Diagram to show the nigro-striatal pathway.

Features of Parkinson's disease

The three *main* features of Parkinson's disease are:
1 *tremor:*
 - present at rest;
 - reduced or eliminated by movement;
 - rhythmic;
 - in hands, legs, tongue, lips and lightly closed eyes;
2 *rigidity:*
 - throughout the full range of movement of individual joints;
 - lead-pipe or cogwheel in quality;
 - present in limbs, trunk and neck;
3 *bradykinesia* (i.e. slowness and poverty of movement):
 - gaze and blinking;
 - facial movement;
 - quiet, monotonous voice and poorly articulated speech;
 - eating and swallowing;
 - hands and fingers for fine manipulative tasks, such as writing and dressing;
 - trunk for turning, either in bed or when walking;
 - legs, making the gait slow and shuffling.

Each of these three features may occur in isolation or in any combination, unilaterally, asymmetrically or bilaterally. The tremor is obvious, well known, publicly identified with Parkinson's disease and an embarrassment. The bradykinesia and rigidity are less overt but much more disabling. This explains the frequency of the most common symptoms of patients with Parkinson's disease:
 - in three-quarters of patients:
   walking slowly;
   slower dressing;
 - in two-thirds of patients:
   difficulty getting out of a chair;
   difficulty turning in bed;
   shuffling;
   stooping when walking;
   speech difficulty;
   difficulty starting movements;
   handwriting change;
 - in one-half of patients:
   tremor.

In addition to the slowness and shuffling of gait, parkinsonian patients may have difficulty in starting to walk. They often shuffle badly in confined spaces and when turning. They occasionally have difficulty in stopping walking (festination), and later in the illness they may have a marked tendency to fall. The falling is in part a consequence of rigidity and akinesia of limb and trunk muscles, but in part due to a failure of more complex postural righting reflex movements.

Since more patients have started to survive longer with Parkinson's disease it has become apparent that later in the illness, memory impairment, confusion, disorientation and other features of dementia are not at all infrequent. This may correspond with observed loss of cholinergic neurones in brainstem nuclei in patients with Parkinson's disease, nuclei that form part of the ascending cholinergic projections to the cerebral cortex, known to be important in patients with dementia.

Management of patients with Parkinson's disease

The management of patients with Parkinson's disease requires sensitivity and patience. The patient is often self-conscious, disappointed, apprehensive and frustrated. He may be more definitely and unequivocally depressed. He is slow to get into the consultation room, sometimes unclear in his speech, slow in undressing for physical examination and frequently keen to discuss 'minor' aspects of his illness, such as constipation. Drug schedules should be altered gradually. Later in the illness, side-effects from the drugs are extremely common, making regular consultations important. As the illness evolves, drug schedules can become quite complicated, needing clear explanation to patient and spouse, especially if some degree of dementia is present in the patient.

Formal physiotherapy is not very helpful for patients with Parkinson's disease. Sticks, walking frames and wheelchairs can be very helpful later on in the illness.

The main form of treatment that helps patients with Parkinson's disease is L-dopa. This is absorbed from the gut, crosses the blood–brain barrier and is converted to dopamine in the brain by the enzyme dopa-decarboxylase. Occasionally, it is given by itself, but more usually it is given with a dopa-decarboxylase inhibitor which does not penetrate the blood–brain barrier. In this way, dopamine levels are not elevated elsewhere in the body (ridding the patient of side-effects due to this, particularly nausea and vomiting), yet the drug is fully active in the brain. Most, but not all, patients respond to L-dopa therapy given in this way. The response may become less complete and/or less long-lived after each dose, as the underlying illness progresses. Larger or more frequently administered doses may be required. Elevation of the dopamine levels in the corpus striatum not infrequently induces choreo-athetoid involuntary movements, and this commonly becomes more evident as the illness progresses. In some patients, the change from the immobile parkinsonian state to the mobile but choreoathetoid state, and back again, in relation to individual doses of L-dopa plus inhibitor can be quite sudden, the so-called 'on-off' phenomenon.

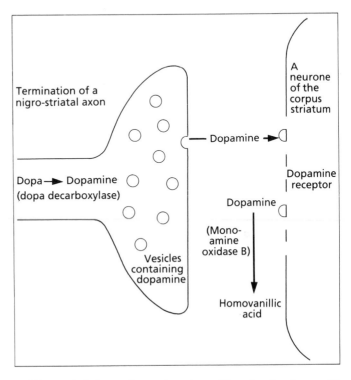

Fig. 9.4. Diagram to show the termination of the nigro-striatal pathway in the corpus striatum.

Figure 9.4 shows how elevation of levels of L-dopa will increase the supply of dopamine to excite dopamine receptors on the surface of the corpus striatum neurones. It also makes it clear why dopamine agonists, e.g. bromocriptine, may be used in Parkinson's disease to stimulate the dopamine receptors directly. Some of the dopamine released by the nigro-striatal neurones will be taken up by the presynaptic terminal for re-use. Some will be transformed to homovanillic acid by the action of mono-amine oxidase type B. Mono-amine oxidase type B inhibitors, e.g. selegiline, will increase the life of released dopamine, and for this reason they are also used in Parkinson's disease. Sometimes, dopamine agonists or mono-amine oxidase type B inhibitors can help a patient whose Parkinson's disease cannot be satisfactorily controlled by medication with L-dopa plus inhibitor.

Anticholinergic therapy, by re-dressing the balance of acetylcholine and dopamine in the corpus striatum (Fig. 9.3), is sometimes of some help to patients with Parkinson's

111   *Tremor and involuntary movement*

disease. Amantadine, which may block re-uptake of dopamine by the presynaptic terminal, is rarely of significant benefit.

In patients in whom tremor is the predominant symptom, a stereotactically induced surgical lesion in the ventrolateral nucleus of the thalamus offers surprisingly good results. The surgery is extremely delicate and somewhat empirical, but carries little risk in capable experienced hands. The ideal candidate for such treatment is a young patient, with severe unilateral tremor in the non-dominant limbs, who has not been helped by drug therapy.

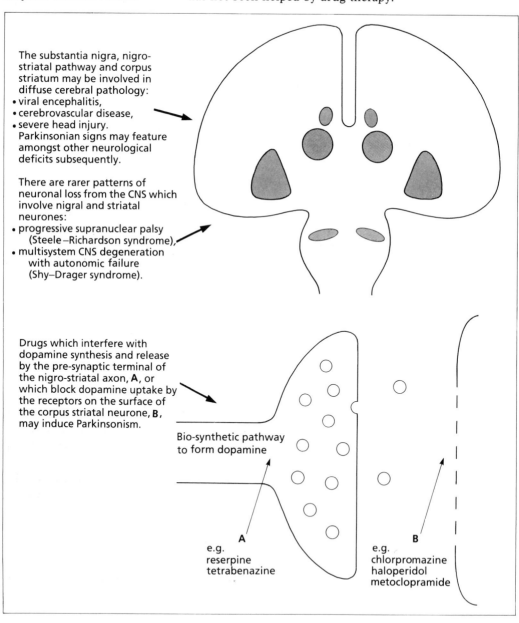

Fig. 9.5. Parkinsonism other than idiopathic Parkinson's disease.

The substantia nigra, nigro-striatal pathway and corpus striatum may be involved in diffuse cerebral pathology:
• viral encephalitis,
• cerebrovascular disease,
• severe head injury.
Parkinsonian signs may feature amongst other neurological deficits subsequently.

There are rarer patterns of neuronal loss from the CNS which involve nigral and striatal neurones:
• progressive supranuclear palsy (Steele–Richardson syndrome),
• multisystem CNS degeneration with autonomic failure (Shy–Drager syndrome).

Drugs which interfere with dopamine synthesis and release by the pre-synaptic terminal of the nigro-striatal axon, **A**, or which block dopamine uptake by the receptors on the surface of the corpus striatal neurone, **B**, may induce Parkinsonism.

Bio-synthetic pathway to form dopamine

A
e.g.
reserpine
tetrabenazine

B
e.g.
chlorpromazine
haloperidol
metoclopramide

Other types of parkinsonism

Other types of parkinsonism are featured in Fig 9.5. The most important, in numerical terms, is drug-induced parkinsonism, which is common in psychiatric patients taking neuroleptic agents that block dopamine receptors in the brain. Very occasionally, this can be very severe and life-threatening, the so-called neuroleptic malignant syndrome.

If a parkinsonian patient shows no response to therapy with L-dopa plus inhibitor, one should question whether the patient has ordinary Parkinson's disease, or whether he has one of the rarer multisystem CNS neuronal degenerations that look somewhat like idiopathic Parkinson's disease.

Chorea, athetosis, dystonia, hemiballismus, tics, myoclonus

Attempted definitions

Chorea: sudden jerking movements which are entirely random in their timing and in their distribution about the body.

Athetosis or dystonia: these two words are used to describe movements which are repetitive or sustained, in which writhing and torsion are conspicuous.

Hemiballismus: large-amplitude, proximal, sudden movements affecting one side of the body.

Tics: repetitive, stereotyped, sudden movements under partial voluntary control.

Myoclonus: brief, shock-like, involuntary muscle jerks.

In this group of movement disorders, there is considerable overlap in clinical practice. For example, the involuntary movements generated by L-dopa in patients with Parkinson's disease are generally referred to as choreo-athetoid, since they have features of chorea and athetosis. As another example, the unilateral involuntary movements of hemiballismus may be quite small in amplitude and gentle, in which case the patient may be said to be suffering from hemichorea.

None of the disorders is very common, with the possible exception of the drug-induced states, so none will be described in great detail.

Drug-induced movement disorders

We have seen already how *tremor* and *parkinsonism* can be induced by drugs, and we will see later in the chapter how *cerebellar ataxia* may also be the result of drugs.

Choreo-athetoid and dystonic movements may be encountered with drugs known to have a pharmacological action in the basal ganglia:

• in patients with Parkinson's disease *L-dopa plus inhibitor, dopamine agonists and MAO type B inhibitors* commonly induce choreo-athetoid involuntary movements;

• *phenothiazines, haloperidol, and metoclopramide* can all cause acute dystonia in which there are spasmodic contractions, in one or more muscle groups. Oculo-gyric crisis, trismus, torticollis, and opisthotonus may all occur;

• in patients with schizophrenia, long-term use of *neuroleptic drugs* may induce involuntary movements around the mouth and face, and occasionally widespread dystonia. This is known as tardive dyskinesia.

Athetosis in brain-damaged children from birth

Athetoid movements and dystonic postures may occur as part of the evidence of damage to the brain around the time of birth. The patient may have a low IQ, suffer from epilepsy, and have other neurological deficits as other evidence of the same insult, but not necessarily so. Kernicterus, as a consequence of inadequately managed rhesus incompatibility problems in the neonatal period, is particularly likely to result in athetoid movements.

Huntington's chorea

This is a progressive hereditary disorder characterized by loss of cells from the basal ganglia and cerebral cortex, giving rise to progressive chorea, dementia and behavioural changes. It is inherited by an autosomal dominant gene, and a genetic marker for the presence of this gene is now established. Predictive statements about young and unborn offspring of patients with the condition will soon be possible as a routine clinical service, with all the ethical problems that surround the availability of such a test.

In terms of basal ganglion function, Huntington's chorea and Parkinson's disease are polar opposites.

1 Dopaminergic drugs:
  • improve Parkinson's disease but may induce choreo-athetoid involuntary movements;
  • worsen the chorea of Huntington's patients.

2 Drugs inhibiting the synthesis of dopamine, and drugs which block dopamine receptors:
  • worsen patients with Parkinson's disease;
  • induce parkinsonism in psychiatric patients;
  • improve the chorea of Huntington's patients.

Sydenham's chorea

This used to be a common sequel to streptococcal infection in young people, along with rheumatic fever; neither is seen commonly now.

Wilson's disease

This is a rare metabolic disorder characterized by the deposition of copper in various organs of the body, especially brain, liver and ⸌ornea. It is due to an inadequate level of the enzyme, caeruloplasmin, in the body. It is an inherited autosomal recessive condition.

In the brain, it chiefly disturbs basal ganglion function, giving rise to all sorts of movement disorders, though impaired intellectual function and other neurological symptoms and signs may also be evident. In the liver, it may give rise to cirrhosis and failure, and in the cornea it is visible peripherally as the Kayser–Fleischer ring.

Chelating agents, such as penicillamine, are used to leech the copper out of the body. They have certainly altered the outlook for patients with Wilson's disease who are diagnosed early, whilst brain and liver changes are reversible.

Hemiballismus

Usually, in the wake of a vascular lesion involving the subthalamic nucleus on one side, contralateral, large-amplitude, involuntary movements involving proximal muscles may occur. The condition is not common and tends to resolve over a few weeks. It is diminished by dopamine-blocking drugs.

Other involuntary movements

Other rare syndromes in which involuntary movements occur, and where the pathological basis is poorly understood, include:
- *spasmodic torticollis* (involuntary turning of the head to one side);
- *writer's cramp* (involuntary tightening of the fingers, hands and forearm when writing);
- *clonic hemifacial spasm* (involuntary intermittent contraction of the muscles supplied by the facial nerve on one side of the face);
- *blephorospasm* (involuntary sustained closure of both eyes);
- *nervous tics* (repetitive stereotyped movements around the head and shoulders in children, with good prognosis);

115   *Tremor and involuntary movement*

- *myoclonic jerks*. These may occur:

singly in normal people whilst going to sleep, usually in the legs;

as a feature of idiopathic epilepsy, usually in the arms and shortly after waking, in teenagers and young adults;

as infantile spasms, salaam attacks, in infants with a marked epileptic tendency (hypsarrhythmia);

as a permanent, disabling, major interference with any voluntary movement, in some patients surviving cardio-respiratory arrest (post-anoxic action myoclonus);

in a variety of other rare epileptic, degenerative, or metabolic encephalopathies.

Cerebellar ataxia

Figure 9.6 is a grossly oversimplified representation of the cerebellum. The function of the cerebellum is to coordinate agonist, antagonist and synergist muscle activity in the performance of learned movements, and to maintain body equilibrium whilst such movements are being executed. Using a massive amount of input from proprioceptors throughout the body, from the inner ear and from the cerebral hemispheres, a complex subconscious computation occurs within the cerebellum. The product of this process largely re-enters the CNS through the superior peduncle and ensures a smooth and orderly sequence of muscular contraction, characteristic of voluntary skilled movement.

In man, the function of the cerebellum is seen at its best in athletes, sportsmen, gymnasts, and ballet dancers, and at its worst during states of alcoholic intoxication when all the features of cerebellar malfunction appear. A concern of patients with organic cerebellar disease is that people will think they are drunk.

Localization of lesions

From Fig 9.6 it is clear that patients may show defective cerebellar function if they have lesions in the cerebellum itself, in the cerebellar peduncles, or in the midbrain, pons or medulla. The rest of the central nervous system will lack the benefit of correct cerebellar function whether the pathology is in the cerebellum itself, or in its incoming and outflowing connections. Localization of the lesion may be possible on the basis of the clinical signs.

- *Midline cerebellar lesions* predominantly interfere with the maintenance of body equilibrium, producing gait and stance ataxia, without too much ataxia of limb movement.

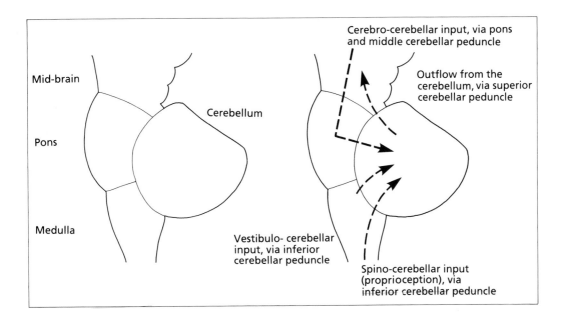

Cerebro-cerebellar input, via pons and middle cerebellar peduncle

Outflow from the cerebellum, via superior cerebellar peduncle

Mid-brain

Cerebellum

Pons

Medulla

Vestibulo- cerebellar input, via inferior cerebellar peduncle

Spino-cerebellar input (proprioception), via inferior cerebellar peduncle

Fig. 9.6. Highly simplified diagrammatic representation of the brainstem and cerebellum as viewed from the left.

• *Lesions in the superior cerebellar peduncle*, along the course of one of the chief outflow tracts from the dentate nucleus in the cerebellum to the red nucleus in the midbrain, classically produce a very marked intention tremor, as mentioned at the beginning of this chapter.

• *Lesions in the midbrain, pons and medulla*, which are causing cerebellar deficits by interfering with inflow or outflow pathways to or from the cerebellum, may also cause other brainstem signs, e.g. cranial nerve palsies, and/or long tract signs (upper motor neurone or sensory) in the limbs.

Clinical signs of cerebellar dysfunction

The common, important clinical signs of cerebellar dysfunction are listed below.

• *Nystagmus.*

• *Dysarthria*: the muscles of voice production and speech lack coordination so that sudden irregular changes in volume and timing occur, i.e. scanning or staccato speech.

• *Upper limbs: ataxia* and *intention tremor*, best seen in movement directed towards a restricted target, e.g. the finger–nose test; *dysdiadokokinesia*, i.e. slow, inaccurate, rapid alternating movements.

• *Lower limbs: ataxia*, best seen in the heel–knee–shin test.

• *Gait and stance ataxia*, especially if the patient is asked to walk heel-to-toe, or to stand still on one leg.

• *Hypotonia*, though a feature of cerebellar lesions, is not very useful in clinical practice.

Cerebellar representation is ipsilateral, so a left cerebellar hemisphere lesion will produce nystagmus which is of greater amplitude when the patient looks to the left, ataxia which is more evident in the left limbs, and a tendency to deviate or fall to the left when standing or walking.

To date, it has not been possible to improve defective cerebellar function pharmacologically.

Causes of cerebellar malfunction

The common causes of cerebellar malfunction are:
- cerebrovascular disease;
- multiple sclerosis;
- drugs, especially anticonvulsant intoxication;
- alcohol, acute intoxication.

Rarer cerebellar lesions include:
- posterior fossa tumours:
  primary malignant tumours in children;
  acoustic neuroma and metastatic tumours in adults;
- cerebellar abscess, usually secondary to otitis media;
- cerebellar degeneration:
  heredofamilial syndromes (Friedreich's ataxia);
  multisystem CNS degenerative disease (olivo-ponto-cerebellar degeneration);
  malignant disease, as a non-metastatic effect;
  chronic alcoholism;
- Arnold–Chiari malformation (in which the cerebellum and medulla are unusually low in relation to the foramen magnum);
- hypothyroidism.

Sensory ataxia

Since proprioception is such an important input to the cerebellum for normal movement, it is of little surprise that when it is lacking ataxia may occur, and that this ataxia may resemble cerebellar ataxia.

Pronounced loss of touch sensation, particularly in the hands and feet, seriously interferes with fine manipulative skills in the hands, and with standing and walking in the case of the feet.

In the presence of such sensory loss, the patient compensates by using his eyes to monitor movement of the hands or feet. This may be partially successful. An important clue that a patient's impaired movement is due to sensory loss is that his clumsiness and unsteadiness are worse in the dark, or at other times when his eyes are closed, e.g. washing his face, having a shower, whilst putting clothes over his head in dressing.

Signs of sensory ataxia

In the hands

- Pseudo-athetosis: the patient is unable to keep his fingers still in the outstretched position. Because of the lack of feedback on hand and finger position, curious postures develop in the outstretched fingers and hands when the eyes are closed.
- Clumsiness of finger movement, e.g. when turning over the pages of a book singly, and when manipulating small objects in the hands, made much worse by eye closure. Shirt and pyjama top buttons, which cannot be seen, present more difficulty than other buttons.
- Difficulty in recognizing objects placed in the hands when the patient's eyes are closed, and difficulty in selecting familiar articles from pockets and hand-bags without the use of the eyes.
- Loss of touch and joint position sense in the fingers.

In the legs

- Marked and unequivocal Rombergism. The patient immediately becomes hopelessly unsteady in the standing position when the eyes are closed.
- As the patient walks, he is obviously looking at the ground and at his feet.
- Loss of touch and joint position sense in the feet and toes.

Causes of sensory ataxia

Sensory ataxia is most commonly encountered in the following circumstances:
- *peripheral neuropathy;*
- *spinal cord disease* interfering with posterior column function. Nowadays, cervical myelopathy, due to cervical spondylosis, and multiple sclerosis are more commonly responsible for this. Subacute combined degeneration of the cord (due to vitamin B_{12} deficiency) and tabes dorsalis (due to tertiary syphilis) are rare;
- *cerebral hemisphere lesions* involving the thalamus or sensory cortex.

Chapter 10   Paraplegia

Anatomical considerations

Figure 10.1 shows the relationship of the spinal cord, dura, spinal nerves and vertebrae to each other. The important points to note are:
• the spinal cord terminates at the level of the L1 vertebra. Any disease process below the level of this vertebra may cause neurological problems, but it will do so by interfering with function in the cauda equina not in the spinal cord;
• because the vertebral column is so much longer than the spinal cord, there is a progressive slip in the numerical value of the vertebra with the numerical value of the spinal cord at that level, e.g.

C8 vertebra corresponds to T1 cord
T10 vertebra corresponds to T12 cord
L1 vertebra corresponds to S1 cord;

• the spinal cord is fatter in the cervical and lumbosacral segments because of upper and lower limb innervation;
• the dural lining of the bony spinal canal runs right down to the sacrum, housing the cauda equina below the level of the spinal cord at L1;
• the vertebrae become progressively more massive because of the increasing weight-bearing load put upon them.

Figure 10.2 is a representation of those tracts in the spinal cord which are important from the clinical point of view:
• the lateral cortico-spinal, or pyramidal, tract from the left hemisphere crosses from left to right in the lower medulla and innervates lower motor neurones in the right ventral horn. Axons from these lower motor neurones in turn innervate muscles in the right arm, trunk and leg;
• the posterior column contains ascending sensory axons carrying proprioception and vibration sense from the right side of the body. These are axons of dorsal root ganglion cells situated beside the right-hand side of the spinal cord. After relay and decussation in the medulla, this pathway gains the left thalamus and left sensory cortex;
• the lateral spino-thalamic tract consists of sensory axons

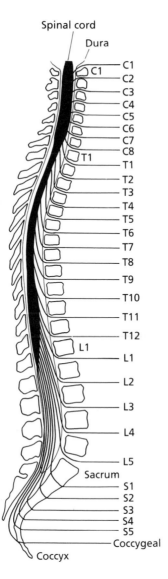

Spinal cord

Dura

C1
C1
C2
C3
C4
C5
C6
C7
C8
T1
T1
T2
T3
T4
T5
T6
T7
T8
T9
T10
T11
T12
L1
L1
L2
L3
L4
L5
Sacrum
S1
S2
S3
S4
S5
Coccygeal
Coccyx

Fig. 10.1. Diagram to show the relationship of the spinal cord, dura and spinal nerves to the vertebrae.

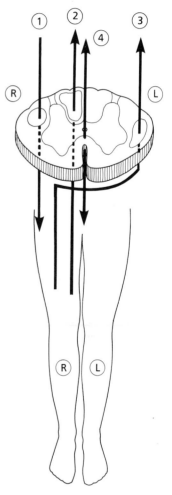

1 = Pyramidal tract

2 = Posterior column

3 = Lateral spino-thalamic tract

4 = Tracts having important autonomic function

Fig. 10.2. Diagram to show the spinal cord, the important tracts and their relationship to the legs.

carrying pain and temperature sense from the right side of the body. These are axons of neurones situated in the right posterior horn of the spinal cord, which decussate and ascend as the spinothalamic tract to gain the left thalamus and left sensory cortex;

• ascending and descending pathways (which are less well-defined tracts, on both sides of the spinal cord) subserving bladder, bowel and sexual function.

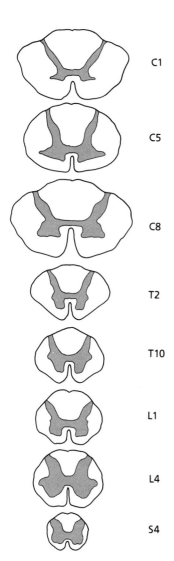

C1

C5

C8

T2

T10

L1

L4

S4

Fig. 10.3. Transverse sections of the spinal cord taken at different levels.

Figure 10.3 shows transverse sections of the spinal cord at various levels. The important points to note are:
• the increased mass of grey matter in the lower cervical and lumbo-sacral regions of the cord, to innervate the limbs;
• the progressive increase in white matter as one passes up the spinal cord due to the increasing expansion of ascending and descending fibre tracts.

Figure 10.4 shows the upper aspect of a cervical vertebra, noting the bony spinal canal, lined by dura, in which the spinal cord lies. Four points are important from the clinical point of view:
• some individuals have wide spinal canals, some have narrow spinal canals. People with constitutionally narrow canals are more vulnerable to cord compression by any mass lesion encroaching upon the spinal cord;
• the vulnerability of the spinal nerve, in or near the intervertebral foramen, (i) to the presence of a posterolateral intervertebral disc protrusion and (ii) to osteoarthritic enlargement of the intervertebral facet joint;
• the vulnerability of the spinal cord, in the spinal canal, to a large posterior intervertebral disc protrusion;
• below the first lumbar vertebra a constitutionally narrow canal will predispose to cauda equina compression.

Clinical considerations

The clinical picture of a patient presenting with a lesion in the spinal cord is a composite of tract signs and segmental signs, as shown in Fig. 10.5.

Tract signs

A *complete* lesion, affecting all parts of the cord at one level (Fig. 10.6), will give rise to:
• bilateral upper motor neurone paralysis of the part of the body below the level of the lesion;
• bilateral loss of all modalities of sensation below the level of the lesion;
• complete loss of all bladder, bowel and sexual function.

It is more frequent for lesions to be *incomplete*, however, and this may be in two ways.
1 The lesion may be affecting all parts of the spinal cord at one level (Fig. 10.6a), but not completely stopping all function in the descending and ascending tracts. In this case there is:
• bilateral weakness, but not complete paralysis, below the level of the lesion;
• impaired sensory function, but not complete loss;

122   *Chapter 10*

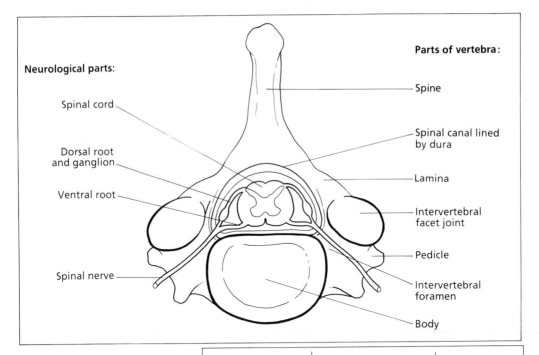

Neurological parts:

Spinal cord

Dorsal root
and ganglion

Ventral root

Spinal nerve

Parts of vertebra:

Spine

Spinal canal lined
by dura

Lamina

Intervertebral
facet joint

Pedicle

Intervertebral
foramen

Body

Fig. 10.4. Superior aspect of a cervical vertebra, showing the spinal cord, the nerve roots, and the spinal nerves.

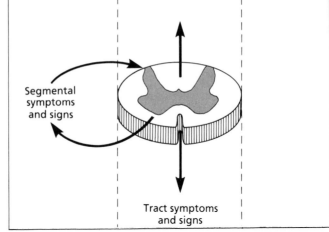

Segmental
symptoms
and signs

Tract symptoms
and signs

Fig. 10.5. Diagram to show that the clinical phenomena generated by a spinal cord lesion are a composite of tract and segmental features.

• defective bladder, bowel and sexual function, rather than complete lack of function.

2 At the level of the lesion, function in one part of the cord may be more affected than elsewhere, for instance:

• just one side of the spinal cord may be affected at the site of the lesion (Fig. 10.6b), the so-called Brown–Seqard syndrome;

• the lesion may be interfering with function in the posterior columns, with little effect on other parts of the cord (Fig. 10.6c);

• the anterior and lateral parts of the cord may be damaged, with relative sparing of posterior column function (Fig. 10.6d).

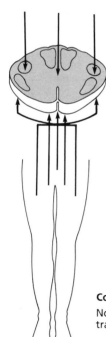

Complete spinal cord lesion

No downward or upward transmission of impulses

(a)

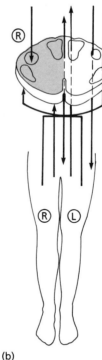

Right sided spinal cord lesion

No neurotransmission in:—

Right pyramidal tract ∴ UMN signs ®️ leg

Right posterior column ∴ position and vibration sense loss ®️ leg

Right spino-thalamic tract ∴ pain and temperature sense loss Ⓛ leg

Effect upon bladder variable, probably just intact

(b)

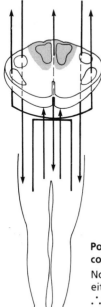

Posterior column spinal cord lesion

No neurotransmission in either posterior column ∴ position and vibration sense loss in both legs Bladder probably intact

(c)

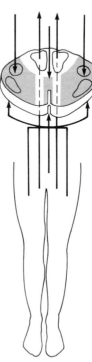

Anterolateral column spinal cord lesion

No neurotransmission in:—

Either pyramidal tracts ∴ UMN signs both legs

Either spino-thalamic tracts ∴ pain and temperature sense loss both legs

Tracts to bladder, bowel etc ∴ incontinence, retention, constipation

(d)

Fig. 10.6 (*opposite*). Diagram to show various spinal cord lesions and their tract signs. (a) A complete spinal cord lesion. (b) A right-sided spinal cord lesion. (c) A posterior spinal cord lesion. (d) An anterolateral spinal cord lesion.

Fig. 10.7. The segmental and tract symptoms and signs of a right-sided C5/6 spinal cord lesion.

The level of the lesion in the spinal cord may be deduced by finding the upper limit of the physical signs due to tract malfunction when examining the patient. For instance, in a patient with clear upper motor neurone signs in the legs, the presence of upper motor neurone signs in the arms is good evidence that the lesion is above C5. If the arms and hands are completely normal on examination, a spinal cord lesion below T1 is more likely.

Segmental signs

In addition to interfering with function in the ascending and descending tracts, a spinal cord lesion may disturb sensory input, reflex activity and lower motor neurone outflow at the level of the lesion. These segmental features may be unilateral or bilateral, depending on the nature of the causative pathology. Chief amongst the segmental symptoms and signs are:
- pain in the spine at the level of the lesion (caused by the pathological causative process);
- pain, paraesthesiae, or sensory loss in the relevant dermatome (caused by involvement of the dorsal nerve root, or dorsal horn, in the lesion);
- lower motor neurone signs in the relevant myotome (caused by involvement of the ventral nerve root, or ventral horn, in the lesion);
- loss of deep tendon reflexes, if reflex arcs which can be assessed clinically are present at the relevant level. (A lesion at C5/6 may show itself in this way by loss of the biceps or supinator jerks. A lesion at C2/3 will not cause loss of deep

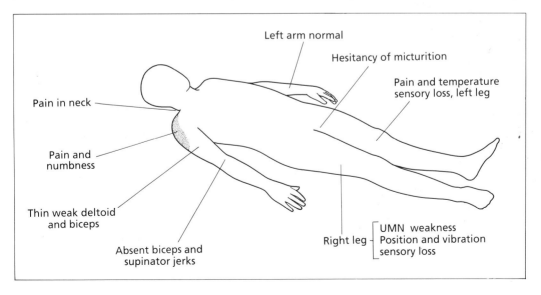

Left arm normal

Hesitancy of micturition

Pain and temperature sensory loss, left leg

Pain in neck

Pain and numbness

Thin weak deltoid and biceps

Absent biceps and supinator jerks

Right leg — UMN weakness / Position and vibration sensory loss tendon reflexes on clinical examination, since stretch reflexes in muscles supplied by these segments cannot be assessed clinically.)

A common example of the value of segmental symptoms and signs in assessing the level of a spinal cord lesion is shown in Fig. 10.7.

Knowledge of all dermatomes, myotomes and reflex arc segmental values is not essential to practise clinical neurology, but some are vital. The essential requirements are shown in Fig. 10.8.

Before proceeding to consider the causes of paraplegia in the next section, two further, rather obvious, points should be noted.

• Paraplegia is commoner than tetraplegia. This is simply a reflection of the fact that there is a much greater length of spinal cord, vulnerable to various diseases, involved in leg innervation (from the foramen magnum to thoracic vertebra T9 or 10) than in arm innervation (from the foramen magnum to the 2nd or 3rd cervical vertebra), as shown in Fig. 10.1.

Fig. 10.8. The important dermatomes, myotomes, and reflex arc segmental values, with which a student should be conversant.

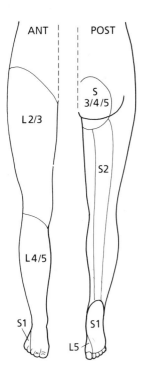

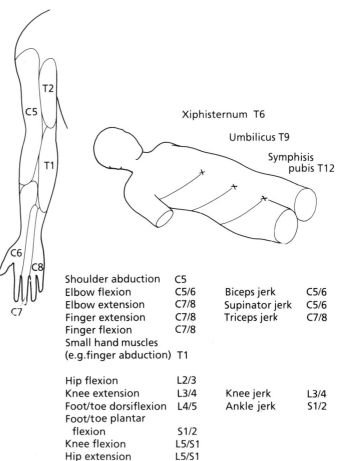

Xiphisternum T6

Umbilicus T9

Symphisis pubis T12

Shoulder abduction	C5		
Elbow flexion	C5/6	Biceps jerk	C5/6
Elbow extension	C7/8	Supinator jerk	C5/6
Finger extension	C7/8	Triceps jerk	C7/8
Finger flexion	C7/8		
Small hand muscles (e.g. finger abduction)	T1		

Hip flexion	L2/3		
Knee extension	L3/4	Knee jerk	L3/4
Foot/toe dorsiflexion	L4/5	Ankle jerk	S1/2
Foot/toe plantar flexion	S1/2		
Knee flexion	L5/S1		
Hip extension	L5/S1		

126 *Chapter 10*

• At the beginning of this section, and in Fig. 10.5, it was stated that patients with spinal cord lesions present with a composite picture of tract and segmental signs. This is the truth, but not the whole truth. It would be more accurate to say that such patients present with the features of their spinal cord lesion (tract and segmental), and with the features of the cause of their spinal cord lesion. At the same time as we are assessing the site and severity of the spinal cord lesion in a patient, we should be looking for clinical clues of the cause of the lesion. This is discussed in the next section.

The causes of paraplegia

The causes of paraplegia are illustrated in Fig. 10.9, with some extra detail about the four common causes of spinal cord dysfunction: trauma, demyelination, malignant disease and spondylotic degenerative disease of the spine. One or two further points will be made about each of these relatively common diseases.

Trauma

Road traffic accidents and falls are the commonest cause, and the order of frequency of injury in terms of neurological level is cervical, then thoracic, then lumbar. Initial care at the site of the accident is vitally important, ensuring that neurological damage is not incurred or increased by clumsy inexperienced movement of the patient at this stage. Unless the life of the patient is in jeopardy by leaving him at the site of the accident, one person should not attempt to move the patient. He should await the arrival of four or five other people, hopefully with a medical or paramedical person in attendance. Movement of the patient suspected of spinal trauma should be slow and careful, with or without the aid of adequate machinery to 'cut' the patient out of distorted vehicles. It should be carried out by several people able to support different parts of the body, so that the patient is moved in one piece.

Demyelination

An episode of paraplegia in a patient with multiple sclerosis usually evolves over the period of 1–2 weeks, as with other episodes of demyelination elsewhere in the CNS. Occasionally, however, the paraplegia may evolve slowly and insidiously (see Chapter 11).

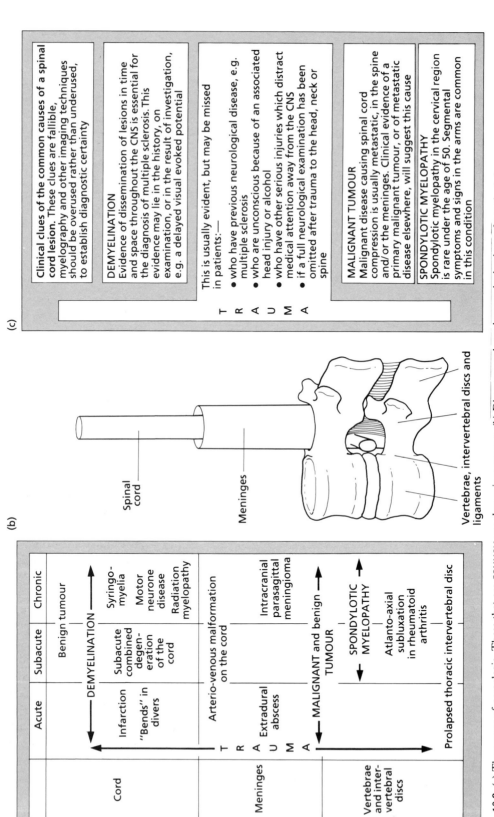

(a)

	Acute	Subacute	Chronic
Cord	← DEMYELINATION →		
	Infarction "Bends" in divers	Benign tumour	
		Subacute combined degeneration of the cord	Syringomyelia Motor neurone disease Radiation myelopathy
Meninges	Arterio-venous malformation on the cord		
	T R A Extradural U abscess M A	← MALIGNANT and benign TUMOUR →	Intracranial parasagittal meningioma
		SPONDYLOTIC MYELOPATHY Atlanto-axial subluxation in rheumatoid arthritis	
Vertebrae and intervertebral discs	Prolapsed thoracic intervertebral disc		

(b)

Spinal cord

Meninges

Vertebrae, intervertebral discs and ligaments

(c)

Clinical clues of the common causes of a spinal cord lesion. These clues are fallible, myelography and other imaging techniques should be overused rather than underused, to establish diagnostic certainty

DEMYELINATION

Evidence of dissemination of lesions in time and space throughout the CNS is essential for the diagnosis of multiple sclerosis. This evidence may lie in the history, on examination, or in the result of investigation, e.g. a delayed visual evoked potential

This is usually evident, but may be missed in patients:—

T
R • who have previous neurological disease, e.g. multiple sclerosis
A • who are unconscious because of an associated head injury or alcohol
U
M • who have other serious injuries which distract medical attention away from the CNS
A • if a full neurological examination has been omitted after trauma to the head, neck or spine

MALIGNANT TUMOUR

Malignant disease causing spinal cord compression is usually metastatic, in the spine and/or the meninges. Clinical evidence of a primary malignant tumour, or of metastatic disease elsewhere, will suggest this cause

SPONDYLOTIC MYELOPATHY

Spondylotic myelopathy in the cervical region is rare under the age of 50. Segmental symptoms and signs in the arms are common in this condition

Fig. 10.9. (a) The causes of paraplegia. Those that are COMMON are shown in CAPITALS. (b) Diagram to show the vertebral column from the left. (c) Clinical clues of the common causes of a spinal cord lesion.

Malignant disease of the spine

Secondary deposits of carcinoma are the main type of trouble in this category; myeloma, lymphoma, leukaemia, sarcoma are all much less common. Often, plain X-rays of the spine will show vertebral deposits within and beside the spine, but sometimes the tumour deposit is primarily meningeal with little bony change. Surgical decompression, radiotherapy or chemotherapy can sometimes make a lot of difference to the disability suffered by such patients, even though their long-term prognosis is poor.

Spondylotic myelopathy

Patients with central posterior intervertebral disc prolapse between C4 and T1, with or without constitutionally narrow canals, make up the majority of this group. The cord compression may be at more than one level. The myelopathy may be compressive or ischaemic in nature (the latter due to interference with arterial supply and venous drainage of the cord in the presence of multiple-level disc degenerative disease in the neck). Decompressive surgery, by posterior laminectomy, is aimed at preventing further deterioration in the patient, rather than guaranteeing improvement.

Rarer causes of spinal cord disease

• *Infarction* is remarkably uncommon as a result of atheroma or embolism compared with the frequency of cerebral ischaemic disease.
• *'Bends'* are due to the development of nitrogen bubbles in the body of divers who leave their compressed environment too fast. The bubbles most commonly afflict joints, skin, brain, spinal cord and lungs. Permanent neurological disability may follow the cerebral or spinal pathology. Urgent recompression and subsequent gradual decompression constitute the early management.
• *Extradural abscess* should be suspected in a patient with a spinal cord lesion who is febrile, especially if he is predisposed to infections, e.g. by diabetes or immuno-suppression.
• *Subacute combined degeneration of the spinal cord* should be suspected if there is anaemia, an elevated mean corpuscular volume, or any evidence of peripheral neuropathy. Serum vitamin B_{12} estimation should be part of the investigation of any patient whose progressive spinal cord lesion defies other obvious explanation.
• *Arterio-venous malformations* on the surface of the spinal cord may cause sudden changes in cord function by virtue of

ischaemia or haemorrhage, or they may cause more gradual evolution of symptoms by acting as cord compressive lesions. They are more common in the lower parts of the spinal cord.

• *Prolapsed intervertebral discs in the thoracic region* are uncommon, and a difficult surgical proposition to remove. The spinal canal is very narrow in the thoracic region.

• *Benign tumours of the spinal cord* are usually low-grade gliomas, difficult to treat by surgery or radiotherapy.

• *Syringomyelia* and *motor neurone disease* are discussed elsewhere, in a later section of this chapter, and in Chapter 14, respectively.

• *Radiation myelopathy* is not common now that such careful planning goes into the preparation of radiotherapy treatment schedules. There is usually a latency of months or years between the exposure to radiation and the development of myelopathy.

• A *parasagittal meningioma* is an occasional cause of leg monoparesis. It is an extremely rare cause of upper motor neurone weakness in both legs.

• The two most frequently encountered extramedullary (outside the spinal cord) benign tumours, which may cause cord compression, are *neurofibroma* (arising from Schwann cells in the nerve roots beside the spinal cord) and *meningioma*. Both are readily treated by surgery.

• *Atlanto-axial subluxation in patients with rheumatoid arthritis* is a major complication in this disease when it occurs. It causes further disability in limbs already disabled by arthritis, and it is difficult to stabilize surgically because of the very soft consistency of vertebrae affected by rheumatoid arthritis.

Management of recently developed undiagnosed paraplegia

Four principles underly the management of patients with evolving paraplegia.
1 'Get on with it!'
2 Care of the patient to prevent unnecessary complications.
3 Establish the diagnosis.
4 Treat the specific cause.

'Get on with it!'

Reversibility is not a conspicuous characteristic of damage to the CNS. It is important to try to establish the diagnosis and treat spinal cord disease whilst the clinical deficit is minor. Recovery from complete cord lesions is slow and imperfect. Hours may make a difference to the outcome of a patient with cord compression.

Care of the patient to prevent unnecessary complications

The parts of the body rendered weak, numb, or functionless by the spinal cord lesion need care. Nurses and physiotherapists are the usual people to provide this.

Skin

- frequent inspection;
- frequent relief of pressure (by turning);
- prevention and vigorous treatment of any damage.

Weak or paralysed limbs

- frequent passive movement and stockings to prevent venous stagnation, thrombosis, and pulmonary embolism;
- frequent passive movement to prevent joint stiffness and contracture, without overstretching;
- exercise of non-paralysed muscles.

Non-functioning bladder and bowels

- catheterization;
- adequate fluids;
- dietary fibre regulation;
- suppositories;
- manual evacuation.

Establish the diagnosis

Foremost in establishing the diagnosis are plain X-rays of the spine, myelography, and other imaging techniques (e.g. CT and MR scans). Many of the causes shown in Fig. 10.9 will be displayed by such techniques.

If the myelogram and other imaging techniques are normal, other investigations may be helpful:
- CSF analysis, visual and spinal evoked potentials — multiple sclerosis;
- EMG studies — motor neurone disease;
- haematological tests and serum vitamin B_{12} estimation — subacute combined degeneration of the cord;
- brain CT scan — parasagittal meningioma.

131 *Paraplegia*

Treat the specific cause

- *Trauma:* spine reduction, alignment and immobilization by operative and non-operative means.
- *Demyelination:* consider use of ACTH.
- *Malignant disease:* surgical decompression, steroids, radiotherapy, chemotherapy.
- *Spondylotic myelopathy:* surgical decompression.
- *Infarction:* nil.
- *Bends:* urgent recompression and gradual decompression.
- *Extradural abscess:* surgery and antibiotics.
- *Subacute combined degeneration of the cord:* vitamin B_{12} injections.
- *Arterio-venous malformation:* embolization or surgery, which may be difficult.
- *Thoracic disc:* surgery, which may be difficult.
- *Benign spinal cord tumours:* nil.
- *Syringomyelia:* consider surgery.
- *Motor neurone disease:* nil.
- *Radiation myelopathy:* nil.
- *Parasagittal meningioma:* surgery, which may be difficult if the sagittal sinus is involved.
- *Spinal neurofibroma and meningioma:* surgery.
- *Atlanto-axial subluxation in rheumatoid arthritis:* consider surgery, which is difficult.

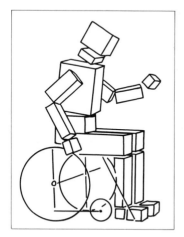

Management of chronic diagnosed paraplegia

From whatever cause, there is a group of patients who have become severely paraplegic, and will remain so on a long-term basis. Their mobility is going to rely heavily on a wheelchair. Multiple sclerosis accounts for the largest number of such patients in the UK, many of whom are young with much of their lives still ahead. Such patients benefit from education, encouragement and the expertise of nurses, physiotherapists, dietitians, social workers, occupational therapists, housing departments, industrial rehabilitation units, psychologists and doctors. They also need the emotional support of their family and friends. They have to come to terms with a major disability and believe in their value despite the loss of normal function in the lower half of their body.

In helping patients to cope with the problem, attention should be given to the following:

1 *Patient education about the level of cord involvement:*

- What does and does not work.

2 *The loss of motor function:*
- wheelchair acceptance and wheelchair skills;
- 'transfers' on and off the wheelchair;
- physiotherapy: passive to prevent joint contractures; active to strengthen non-paralysed muscles.

3 *Sensory loss:*
- care of skin;
- guard against hot, hard or sharp objects;
- taking the weight of the body off the seat of the wheelchair routinely every 15 or 20 minutes.

4 *Bladder:*
- reflex bladder emptying, condom drainage;
- intermittent self-catheterization, indwelling catheter;
- cholinergic or anti-cholinergic drugs as necessary;
- alertness to urinary tract infection.

5 *Bowel:*
- regularity of diet;
- laxatives and suppositories.

6 *Sexual function:*
- often an area of great disappointment;
- normal sexual enjoyment, male ejaculation, orgasm, motor skills for intercourse, all lacking;
- fertility often unimpaired in either sex, though seminal emission in males will require either vibrator stimulation of the fraenum of the penis or electro-ejaculation;
- careful counselling of patient and spouse helps adjustment.

7 *Weight and calories:*
- Wheelchair life probably halves the patient's calorie requirements. It is very easy, and counter-productive, for paraplegic patients to gain weight. Eating and drinking are enjoyable activities left open to them. Heaviness is difficult for their mobility, and bad for the weight-bearing pressure areas.

8 *Psychological aspects:*
- disappointment, depression, shame, resentment, anger, and a sense of an altered role in the family are some of the natural feelings that paraplegic patients experience.

9 *Family support:*
- the presence or absence of this makes a very great difference to the ease of life of a paraplegic patient.

10 *Employment:*
- the patient's self-esteem may be much higher if he can still continue his previous work, or if he can be re-trained to obtain new work.

11 *House adaptation:*
- this is almost inevitable and very helpful. Living on the ground floor, with modifications for a wheelchair life, is important.

12 *Car adaptation:*
- conversion of the controls to arm and hand use may give a great deal of independence.

13 *Financial advice:*
- this will often be needed, especially if the patient is not going to be able to work. Medical social workers are conversant with house conversion, attendance, and mobility allowances.

14 *Recreational activity and holidays:*
- should be actively pursued.

15 *Legal advice:*
- this may be required if the paraplegia was the result of an accident, or if the patient's paraplegia leads to marriage disintegration, which sometimes happens.

16 *Respite care:*
- this may be appropriate to help the patient and/or his relatives. It can be arranged in several different ways, e.g.:
  — admission to a young chronic sick unit for 1–2 weeks, on a planned, infrequent, regular basis;
  — a care attendant lives at the patient's home for 1–2 weeks, whilst the relatives take a holiday.

Syringomyelia

It is worth having a short section of this chapter devoted to syringomyelia because the illness is a neurological 'classic'. It brings together much of what we have learnt about cord lesions, and is grossly over-represented in the clinical part of medical professional examinations. It is a rare condition.

The symptoms and signs are due to an intramedullary (within the spinal cord), fluid-filled cavity extending over several segments of the spinal cord (Fig. 10.10a). The cavity, or syrinx, is most evident in the cervical and upper thoracic cord. There may be an associated Arnold–Chiari malfor-

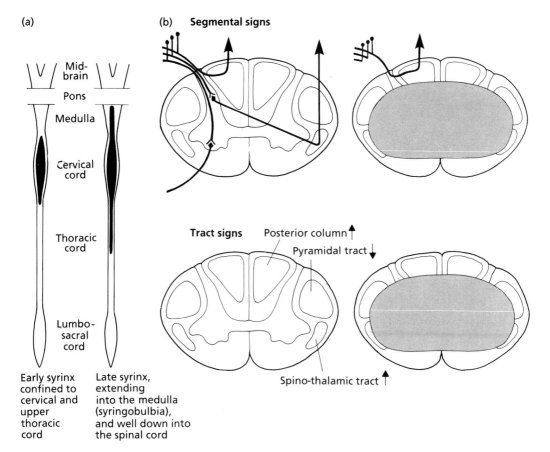

(a)

| Mid-brain |
| Pons |
| Medulla |
| Cervical cord |
| Thoracic cord |
| Lumbo-sacral cord |

(b) **Segmental signs**

Tract signs   Posterior column ↑
                  Pyramidal tract ↓

Spino-thalamic tract ↑

Early syrinx confined to cervical and upper thoracic cord

Late syrinx, extending into the medulla (syringobulbia), and well down into the spinal cord

Fig. 10.10. Diagram to show the main features of syringomyelia. (a) The extent of the cavity in the early and late stages. (b) Segmental and tract signs.

mation at the level of the foramen magnum, in which the medulla and the lowermost parts of the cerebellum are below the level of the foramen magnum. There may be an associated kyphoscoliosis. These associated congenital anomalies suggest that syringomyelia is itself the consequence of malformation of this part of the CNS.

The cavity, and consequent neurological deficit, tend to get larger, very slowly, with the passage of time. This deterioration may occur as sudden exacerbations, between which long stationary periods occur.

The symptoms and signs are the direct consequence of a lesion that extends over several segments within the substance of the cord. There is a combination of segmental and tract signs, as shown in Fig. 10.10b.

Over the length of the cord affected by the syrinx there are segmental symptoms and signs. These are mainly found in the upper limbs, since the syrinx is in the cervical and upper dorsal part of the cord.

• Pain sometimes, but usually transient at the time of an exacerbation.
• Sensory loss which affects pain and temperature, and

135 *Paraplegia*

often leaves posterior column function intact. Burns and poorly healed sores over the skin of the arms are common because of the anaesthesia. The sensory loss of pain and temperature with preserved proprioceptive sense is known as dissociated sensory loss.

• Areflexia, due to the interruption of the monosynaptic stretch reflex within the cord.

• lower motor neurone signs of wasting and weakness.

In the legs, below the level of the syrinx, there may be motor or sensory signs due to descending or ascending tract involvement by the syrinx. Most common of such signs are upper motor neurone weakness, with increased tone, increased reflexes and extensor plantar responses.

Figures 10.10 (a) and (b) are drawn symmetrically, but commonly the clinical expression of syringomyelia is asymmetrical. Painless burns and dissociated anaesthesia in arms and hands that are wasted, weak and areflexic, in a young adult who has a mild spastic paraparesis — this is the distinctive clinical picture of syringomyelia.

Extension of the syrinx into the medulla (syringobulbia), or medullary compression due to the associated Arnold–Chiari malformation, may result in cerebellar and bulbar signs:

• nystagmus and ataxia;

• trigeminal sensory loss on the face;

• dysphagia;

• dysarthria;

• aspiration pneumonia.

The loss of pain sensation in the arms may lead to the development of gross joint disorganization and osteo-arthritic change (described by Charcot) in the upper limbs.

There has been a good deal of theorizing about the mechanisms responsible for the cavity formation within the spinal cord in syringomyelia. No one hypothesis yet stands firm. Certainly, a hydrodynamic abnormality in the region of the foramen magnum may exist in those patients with an Arnold-Chiari malformation, and further deterioration may be prevented by surgical decompression of the lower medullary region in these patients (removal of the posterior margin of the foramen magnum).

Chapter 11

Multiple sclerosis

General comments

After stroke, Parkinson's disease and multiple sclerosis are the two commonest physically disabling diseases of the CNS in the UK. Multiple sclerosis affects young people however, usually presenting between the ages of 20 and 40 years, which is quite different from stroke and Parkinson's disease, which are unusual conditions in patients under 45.

Though potentially a very severe disease, multiple sclerosis does not inevitably lead to disability, wheelchair life, or worse. As with many crippling diseases, the common image of multiple sclerosis is worse than it usually proves to be in practice. This severe image of the disease is not helped by charities (some of which do noble work for research and welfare in multiple sclerosis) who appeal to the public by presenting the illness as a 'crippler' in print, illustration, or in person. A more correct image of the disease has resulted from a greater frankness between patients and neurologists, so that now it is not only patients who have the disease very severely who know their diagnosis. Nowadays, most patients who are suffering from multiple sclerosis know that this is what is wrong with them, and the majority of these patients will be ambulant, working and playing a full role in society. The poor image of the disease leads to considerable anxiety in young women who develop any visual or sensory symptoms from whatever cause, especially if they have some medical knowledge. Most neurologists will see one or more such patients a week, and will have the pleasure of being able to reassure the patients that their symptoms are not indicative of multiple sclerosis.

On the other hand, the disease is common, and enough patients have the disease severely to make multiple sclerosis one of the commonest causes of major neurological disability amongst people under the age of 50 years. Provision for young patients with major neurological disability is not good in this or many other Western 'civilized' countries. There is still plenty that can be done to help patients who have multiple sclerosis severely, and often this is best supervised and coordinated by their doctor.

The lesion

The classical lesion of multiple sclerosis is a plaque of demyelination in the CNS (see Fig. 11.1). This means:
1 the lesion is in the CNS, not the peripheral nervous system, i.e. in the cerebrum, brainstem, cerebellum or spinal cord. It must be remembered that the optic nerve is an outgrowth from the CNS embryologically. This explains

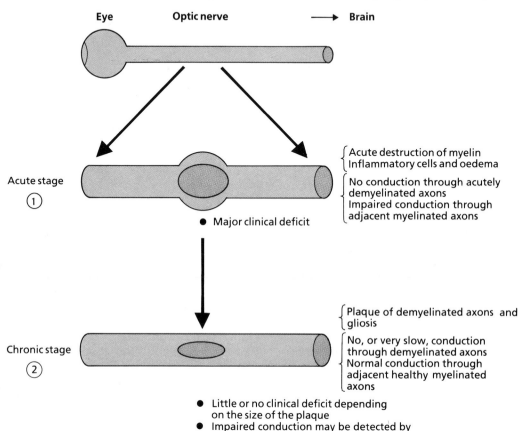

Eye   **Optic nerve**   ⟶   **Brain**

Acute stage
①

{ Acute destruction of myelin
  Inflammatory cells and oedema

{ No conduction through acutely
  demyelinated axons
  Impaired conduction through
  adjacent myelinated axons

● Major clinical deficit

Chronic stage
②

{ Plaque of demyelinated axons and
  gliosis

{ No, or very slow, conduction
  through demyelinated axons
  Normal conduction through
  adjacent healthy myelinated
  axons

● Little or no clinical deficit depending
  on the size of the plaque
● Impaired conduction may be detected by
  sophisticated neurophysiological tests

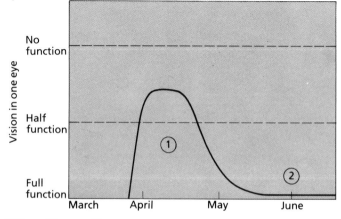

Vision in one eye

No
function

Half
function

Full
function

①

②

March   April   May   June

Fig. 11.1. Diagram to show an episode of demyelination. The optic nerve has been taken as an example in this instance.

why multiple sclerosis frequently involves the optic nerves, whereas lesions in the other cranial nerves, spinal and peripheral nerves in the limbs do not occur;

2 the axons are intact through the lesion, but their myelin sheaths are lost. Saltatory conduction (from node to node along myelinated nerve fibres) cannot occur along the nerve fibres through a plaque of demyelination, and non-saltatory conduction is very slow and inefficient. Neurotransmission is appropriately impaired, depending upon the size of the lesion, for plaques vary considerably in size.

Clinically, the lesion evolves over a few days, lasts for a few days or weeks and gradually settles, as shown in Fig. 11.1. Vision in one eye may deteriorate and improve in this way, or the power in one leg may follow the same pattern. Clearly, the nature of the neurological deficit depends on the site of the plaque of demyelination (in the optic nerve or the pyramidal tract in the spinal cord, in the examples given here).

The evolving pathological lesion underlying the clinical episode is summarized in Fig. 11.1.

Dissemination of lesions in time and place

Multiple sclerosis is caused by the occurrence of lesions just described in different parts of the CNS, occurring at different times in a person's life. This dissemination of lesions in time and place remains the classical and diagnostic characteristic of multiple sclerosis from the clinical point of view.

Lesions may occur anywhere in the CNS. Individual plaques vary in size. The way in which a permanent ongoing disability may evolve in a patient with multiple sclerosis is illustrated in Fig. 11.2, and the common sites of lesions which may occur irregularly during the patient's life are illustrated in Fig. 11.3.

Fig. 11.2. The establishment of a neurological deficit in the right leg by episodes of demyelination along the course of the cortico-spinal tract over a period of 15 years in a patient with multiple sclerosis.

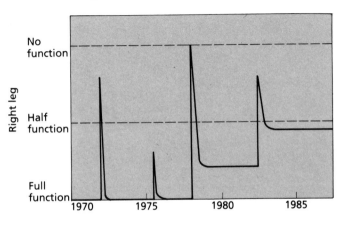

139 *Multiple sclerosis*

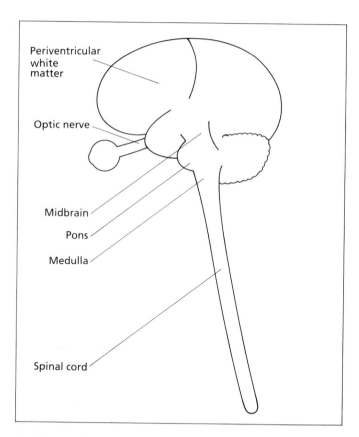

Periventricular
white
matter

Optic nerve

Midbrain

Pons

Medulla

Spinal cord

Fig. 11.3. Diagram to show the common sites at which plaques occur in the CNS of patients with multiple sclerosis.

The number of lesions that show themselves as attacks or relapses in the clinical history of a patient with multiple sclerosis is much less than the number of lesions that can be found in the patient's CNS post-mortem. This agrees with the fact that magnetic resonance imaging of the CNS after the first clinical episode of demyelination frequently shows the presence of plaques elsewhere in the CNS, especially in the periventricular white matter. Furthermore, it is not uncommon to be able to detect lesions in optic, auditory, sensory and motor CNS pathways by electrical neurophysiological techniques in patients with multiple sclerosis. Often, there are no symptoms or signs accompanying such lesions, indicating unsuspected subclinical involvement of various parts of the CNS.

This multiplicity of clinically minor lesions probably explains the gradual (no relapse and remission) type of progression in neurological deficit that may occur in some patients with multiple sclerosis.

Common clinical expressions of multiple sclerosis

This section describes what occurs during individual episodes of demyelination in different parts of the CNS. It also describes the common neurological deficits that characterize a patient who has multiple sclerosis moderately severely. Figure 11.3 shows the common sites for plaques of demyelination.

Periventricular white matter

Lesions are very common in this part of the brain. They are seen early in the disease in patients studied by nuclear magnetic resonance, and are always found post-mortem. They do not give rise to definite symptomatology however, unless they play a part in the impairment of cognitive function, euphoria and emotional lability, which sometimes become apparent in patients who have multiple sclerosis very severely.

Periventricular plaques are common therefore, but not of much apparent clinical importance.

Optic nerve

Optic neuritis is a common and typical manifestation of multiple sclerosis. If the lesion is in the optic nerve between the globe of the eye and the optic chiasm, it is sometimes called retrobulbar (behind the globe of the eye) neuritis. If it is right at the front of the optic nerve, the lesion itself is visible ophthalmoscopically, and is sometimes called papillitis (inflammation of the optic disc). The effect on vision is the same whether the lesion is anterior or posterior in the optic nerve. If anterior, the optic disc is visibly red and swollen, with exudates and haemorrhages. If posterior, the appearance of the optic disc is normal at the time of active neuritis. A section of the optic nerve is acutely inflamed in all instances of optic neuritis, so that pain in the orbit on eye movement is a common symptom.

The effect on vision in the affected eye is to reduce acuity, cause blurring, and this most commonly affects central vision. The patient develops a central scotoma of variable size and density. Colour vision becomes faded, even to a point of fairly uniform greyness. In severe optic neuritis, vision may be lost except for a rim of preserved peripheral vision, or vision may be lost altogether. At this stage, there is a diminished pupil reaction to direct light with a normal consensual response (often called an afferent pupillary defect).

After days or weeks, recovery commences. Recovery from optic neuritis is characteristically very good, taking 4–8 weeks to occur. Five years later, the patient often has difficulty remembering which eye was affected. Occasionally, recovery is slow and incomplete.

The tell-tale signs of a previous episode of optic neuritis may be:
- nothing at all;
- slightly impaired colour vision;
- slightly impaired visual acuity;
- a very mild afferent pupillary defect, when compared with the unaffected other eye;
- a slightly pale optic disc;
- vision that does not seem to be quite normal, even though measured visual acuity, fields and colour vision seem normal;
- vision that becomes impaired by exercise, or by the heat of a hot bath;
- delay in the visual evoked potential. If the cortical responses to monocular visual stimulation are recorded from the occipital region, a delay in neurotransmission through the affected optic nerve can be detected when compared with known normal values.

Midbrain, pons and medulla

Episodes of demyelination in this part of the CNS may cause:
- double vision due to individual cranial nerve dysfunction within the midbrain or pons, or more commonly due to a lesion in the fibre pathways that maintain conjugate movement of the eyes. Lesions of the medial longitudinal fasciculus cause an internuclear ophthalmoplegia, in which there is failure of movement of the adducting eye with preserved movement of the abducting eye, on attempted conjugate deviation of the eyes to one side (see Chapter 12, page 156);
- facial numbness (cranial nerve 5 within the pons);
- facial weakness (cranial nerve 7 within the pons);
- vertigo, nausea, vomiting, ataxia (cranial nerve 8 within the pons);
- dysarthria and occasional dysphagia (cranial nerves 9, 10 and 12 within the medulla);
- cerebellar dysfunction due to lesions on fibre pathways passing in and out of the cerebellum in the cerebellar peduncles, hence nystagmus, dysarthria, ataxia of limbs and gait;
- motor deficits of upper motor neurone type in any of the four limbs;
- sensory deficits, spino-thalamic or posterior column in type, in any of the four limbs.

Spinal cord

Lower motor neurone and segmental signs are unusual in multiple sclerosis. Episodes of demyelination in the spinal cord cause fibre tract (upper motor neurone, posterior column, spinothalamic and autonomic) symptoms and signs below the level of the lesion. Since the length of the fibre tracts in the spinal cord are physically longer for leg function than for arm function, there is a greater likelihood of plaques in the spinal cord interfering with the legs than the arms. Episodes of spinal cord demyelination may cause:

• heaviness, dragging or weakness of the arms, trunk or legs;
• loss of pain and temperature sensation in the arms, trunk or legs;
• tingling, numbness, sense of coldness, sense of skin wetness, sense of skin tightness, or a sensation like that which follows a local anaesthetic or a nettle-sting, in the arms, trunk or legs;
• clumsiness of a hand due to loss of position sense and stereognosis (this particular deficit is more common in the upper limb);
• bladder, bowel or sexual malfunction.

Fig. 11.4. Diagram to show the classical dissemination of lesions in time and space, and the accumulation of a neurological deficit, in a patient who has multiple sclerosis moderately severely.

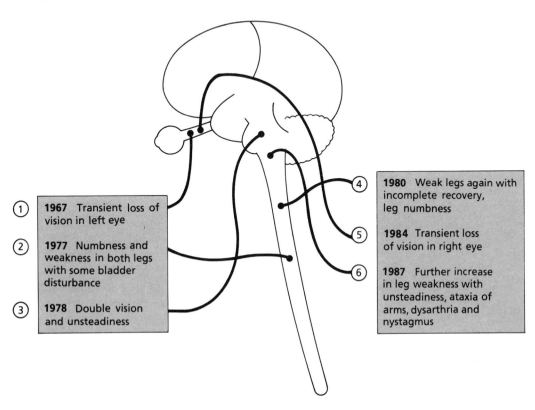

① **1967** Transient loss of vision in left eye

② **1977** Numbness and weakness in both legs with some bladder disturbance

③ **1978** Double vision and unsteadiness

④ **1980** Weak legs again with incomplete recovery, leg numbness

⑤ **1984** Transient loss of vision in right eye

⑥ **1987** Further increase in leg weakness with unsteadiness, ataxia of arms, dysarthria and nystagmus

In a *patient with established multiple sclerosis*, who has suffered multiple episodes of demyelination throughout the CNS (see Fig. 11.4), the accumulated ongoing neurological deficit is likely to consist of:
• asymmetrical optic pallor without a major defect in visual acuity;
• a cerebellar deficit causing nystagmus, dysarthria and arm ataxia;
• an upper motor neurone deficit which is mild in the arms, moderate in the trunk and most evident in the legs. The weakness of the legs often does not allow ataxia to reveal itself in leg movement and walking;
• impaired sexual, bladder and bowel function;
• a variable amount and variety of sensory loss, which is usually more evident in the legs and lower trunk than in the arms.

Uncommon clinical aspects of multiple sclerosis

1 Some patients with multiple sclerosis find that their neurological deficit may be aggravated by the heat of a hot bath, hot weather, or by exercise.
2 Patients with multiple sclerosis affecting the cervical spinal cord may complain of transient electric pins and needles down their arms, back, and legs on neck flexion (L'Hermitte's sign).
3 Patients with multiple sclerosis affecting the brainstem may suffer from trigeminal neuralgia, which behaves just like idiopathic trigeminal neuralgia. It responds to carbamazepine.
4 Patients with multiple sclerosis may suffer from two other paroxysmal transient symptoms: tonic unilateral spasms of the limbs, and episodes of brainstem dysfunction typified by dysarthria and ataxia. The episodes may occur many times a day and can be stopped by carbamazepine.
5 Like anybody else with severe spinal cord disease, patients with severe multiple sclerosis may suffer from flexor or extensor spasms of the legs. These spasms are not usually painful but are a nuisance during movement of the patient. They can be suppressed by baclofen and dantrolene. All the problems attendant upon chronic paraplegia (see Chapter 10) may occur in severely disabled multiple sclerosis patients. Prevention of pressure sores is particularly worthwhile, since healing may require prolonged hospitalization.
6 Some patients' multiple sclerosis is not characterized by the classical relapses and remissions. Some patients seem to get worse, without remission, either in a smoothly progressive way or in a stepwise way.

7 Some patients may suffer a single episode of optic neuritis in one eye, and have no further clinical manifestation of multiple sclerosis. This may happen with an episode of demyelination anywhere in the CNS. The percentage of patients with a single episode of optic neuritis who subsequently go on to develop clinical evidence of multiple sclerosis varies from series to series in the literature. It partly depends on the length of follow-up, but may also depend upon the presence or absence of aetiologically important genetic factors in the patient (e.g. HLA type).

8 One particular pattern of multiple sclerosis consists of the development of bilateral optic neuritis and a spinal cord lesion within the space of 2–3 months. There may or may not be subsequent evidence of active disease in such patients. This pattern of illness is known as neuromyelitis optica or Devic's disease.

Diagnosis

There is no specific laboratory test that confirms the presence of multiple sclerosis. The diagnosis is a clinical one, based upon the occurrence of lesions in the CNS which are disseminated in time and place. Early in the illness it may not be possible to establish the diagnosis therefore, and multiple sclerosis must be held as a possibility whilst other disease processes are eliminated by investigation.

The presence of subclinical lesions in the CNS may be detected by:

• various clinical neurophysiological techniques. Such techniques essentially measure conduction in a CNS pathway, detecting any delay in neurotransmission by comparison with normal control data. Visual, auditory and somatosensory evoked potentials are in regular clinical use for this purpose, as is the measurement of central motor conduction velocity (recording the speed of conduction in the corticospinal tract after magnetic stimulation of the motor cortex);

• imaging techniques. Occasionally, contrast-enhanced brain CT scanning reveals multiple lesions, and frequently MR brain scanning reveals multiple lesions, especially in the periventricular regions.

It must be remembered that delayed CNS conduction and multiple lesions displayed by imaging techniques are not only found in multiple sclerosis. Other disease processes can produce such findings, which must always be assessed in relation to the clinical phenomena occurring in the individual patient.

The inflammatory nature of the demyelinating lesion may result in an elevated lymphocyte count and globulin

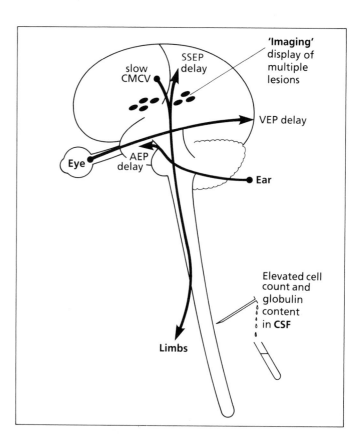

Fig. 11.5. Diagram to show the abnormal investigations in patients with multiple sclerosis.

content in the CSF. These changes also lack specificity. Many other conditions elevate both these parameters. Attempts have been made to fractionate the CSF globulin to produce diagnostic confirmatory evidence of multiple sclerosis. Immuno-electrophoretic demonstration of oligoclonal bands in the CSF globulin has come closest to becoming a diagnostic feature of multiple sclerosis, but it is not specific, producing both false-positive and false-negative results.

Figure 11.5 shows the various abnormal investigations that may be found in patients with multiple sclerosis. None is specific. In suspected cases, the more of these investigations which prove positive, the more likely the diagnosis becomes. It is not surprising that most of these investigations are more positive later on in the illness, when there is no longer any clinical doubt of the diagnosis of multiple sclerosis.

Aetiology

The cause of multiple sclerosis remains unknown.

There appears to be an interaction of an environmental factor with some form of genetically determined patient susceptibility.

The evidence for *genetic susceptibility* is as follows:
- multiple sclerosis is more common in females than males, ratio 1.5:1;
- there is a firm association of multiple sclerosis with certain HLA types, particularly DR2;
- there is an increased incidence of multiple sclerosis in close relatives, about tenfold in first-degree relatives;
- multiple sclerosis is more common in identical than non-identical twins.

The evidence for an *environmental factor* is as follows:
- multiple sclerosis is more common in temperate than in equatorial parts of the world. Migrants moving from high-risk to low-risk areas (e.g. northern Europe to Israel) under the age of puberty acquire low risk;
- higher dietary consumption of animal fat occurs in high-risk areas. Brains of patients with multiple sclerosis contain a higher proportion of saturated fatty acids than controls. It is known that brain lipid composition can be altered by the fatty acid composition of the diet;
- IgG levels are higher in the CSF of patients with multiple sclerosis. Antibodies to measles virus, and to some other viruses, are higher in the CSF of patients with multiple sclerosis.

From these data it is possible to *speculate* about the aetiology of multiple sclerosis:
- some environmental agent (probably infective) gains access to the genetically susceptible person before puberty;
- subsequently there is disease activity affecting myelin in the CNS at variable intervals throughout the patient's adult life;
- the disease activity may represent a continuing interaction between patient and the environmental agent [e.g. latent viral infection within the CNS which occasionally becomes active, as in Herpes simplex (cold sore) and Herpes zoster (shingles) infections];
- alternatively, the disease activity may reflect a state of auto-immunity within the patient, initiated by an abnormal immunological response to the agent at the time of original infection.

147 *Multiple sclerosis*

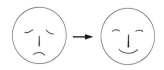

Management

Mild or early cases

1 Inform the patient and family of the diagnosis.
2 Educate the patient and family about multiple sclerosis.
3 Dispel the concept of inevitable progression to major disability.
4 Encourage normal attitudes to life, and normal activities. (This advice should be given initially by the consultant neurologist, and two interviews at an interval will nearly always be needed. Subsequent counselling and support by the family doctor may be very valuable, depending on the patient's reaction to the problem.)

More serious cases

1 Continued education about the nature of multiple sclerosis.
2 Continued support over the disappointment and uncertainty of having multiple sclerosis.
3 Attention to individual symptoms:
  • *vision*, rarely a major problem. Low visual acuity aids may prove helpful in the minority of patients who need them;
  • *cerebellar deficit*, difficult to help. Gross ataxia and intention tremor in an arm may be helped by stereotactic ventrolateral thalamotomy;
  • *paraplegia*, advice as in Chapter 10, page 132.
4 Help from nurses, physiotherapists, occupational therapists, speech therapists, medical social workers, as required.
5 Respite care arrangements, as required.

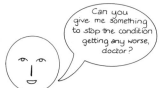

All cases of multiple sclerosis

1 To date, no specific treatment exists for multiple sclerosis.
2 ACTH injections for 3 – 4 weeks reduce the duration and severity of individual episodes of demyelination, without influencing the final outcome.
3 Dietary exclusions and supplements are of no proven advantage. The main dietary requirement is the avoidance of obesity in the enforced sedentary state.
4 Other forms of treatment which have been shown to be of no proven long-term value include:
  • hyperbaric oxygen therapy;
  • spinal cord stimulation;
  • various immuno-suppressive regimes.

Chapter 12   Cranial nerve disorders

Introduction

Disorders of the cranial nerves usually produce clear abnormalities, apparent to both patient and doctor alike. The specialists who become involved in the management of patients with cranial nerve problems are neurologists, neurosurgeons, ophthalmologists (cranial nerves 2–4, 6), dentists (cranial nerve 5), and ENT surgeons (cranial nerves 1, 5, 7–10, 12).

The pattern of involvement of cranial nerves varies from one clinical problem to another, e.g.:
- failure of one cranial nerve on one side, e.g. Bell's palsy;
- failure of one particular cranial nerve on both sides, e.g. methyl alcohol poisoning resulting in bilateral optic nerve damage;
- failure of adjacent cranial nerves on one side because of a local compressive lesion, e.g. 5, 7 and 8 malfunction in the presence of a cerebello-pontine angle tumour (such as an acoustic neuroma);
- failure of several cranial nerves on both sides, e.g. bulbar (5, 7, 9, 10, 12) involvement in motor neurone disease.

Cranial nerves 1, 2, and 11 are a little different from the others. Nerves 1 and 2 are highly specialized extensions of the brain, for smell and sight, in the anterior cranial fossa and suprasellar region. Nerve 11 largely originates from the cervical spinal cord, rises into the posterior fossa only to exit it again very quickly, to supply muscles of the neck and shoulder.

When considering the other cranial nerves, i.e. 3–10 and 12 (as shown in Fig. 12.1), it is useful to remember that the lesion causing malfunction may be nuclear (within the substance of midbrain, pons and medulla), it may be a lesion which is damaging the axons travelling to or from the nucleus still within the substance of the brainstem, or the lesion may be at some point along the course of the nerve, between the surface of the brainstem and the structure which the nerve supplies. Cranial nerve palsies, which are the consequence of intramedullary lesions (within the

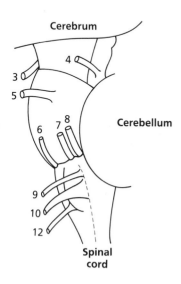

Fig. 12.1 Lateral aspect of the brainstem, and cranial nerves 3–10 and 12 (*seen from the left*).

149   *Cranial nerve disorders*

substance of the brainstem), are commonly associated with long tract signs in the limbs and cerebellar dysfunction, since these are other functions occurring within midbrain, pons and medulla. More peripherally situated cranial nerve lesions have other associations depending upon their position, e.g.:

• visual loss plus pituitary malfunction suggests a lesion in the suprasellar region;

• 3, 4, 5a, and 6 combined malfunction on one side suggests a lesion on the lateral wall of the cavernous sinus;

• severe earache, deafness and facial palsy suggest a lesion in the middle ear cavity.

In this chapter, we will consider the common clinical syndromes associated with each cranial nerve in turn, 1–12.

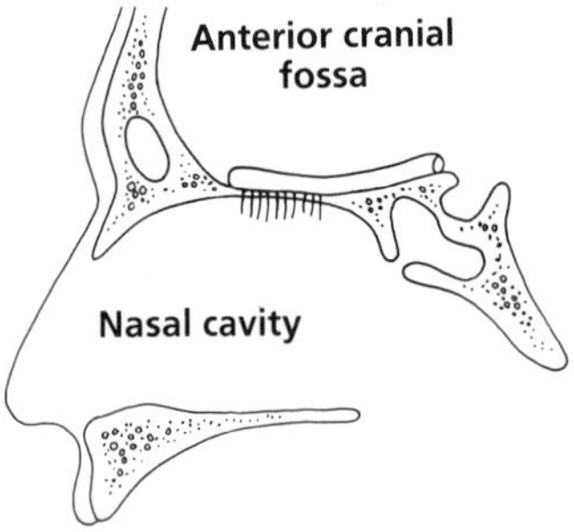

Fig. 12.2. Olfactory nerve and bulb on the floor of the anterior cranial fossa, and olfactory nerve bundles penetrating the thin cribiform plate to innervate the mucosa in the roof of the nasal cavity.

Olfactory nerve (Fig. 12.2)

Patients who have no olfactory function complain of inability to smell or taste. This reflects the fact that subtle taste perception, i.e. that which is more discriminating than sweet, salt, acid or bitter, is achieved by aromatic stimulation of the olfactory nerves in the nose. Patients complain that they are unable to smell, and that all their food tastes the same.

The commonest cause of this loss is nasal obstruction, by infective or allergic oedema of the nasal mucosa. Olfactory nerve lesions are not common. They may result from head injury, either involving fracture in the floor of the anterior fossa, or as a result of damage to the nerves on the rough floor of the anterior fossa at the time of impact of the head injury. Sometimes, the olfactory nerves stop working on a permanent basis for no apparent reason, i.e. idiopathic anosmia. Very occasionally, a tumour arising from the floor of the anterior fossa (e.g. meningioma) may cause unilateral or bilateral loss of olfactory function.

Optic nerve, chiasm, and radiation (Fig. 12.3)

We will now consider the symptoms and signs of the commoner disorders which affect the visual pathways.

Migraine

During the early phases of a migraine attack, when there is vasospasm in some of the cranial arteries, varying neurological or ophthalmological symptoms may occur because of transient ischaemia. Such symptoms rarely last for more than 30 minutes and completely recover. As they are

150   *Chapter 12*

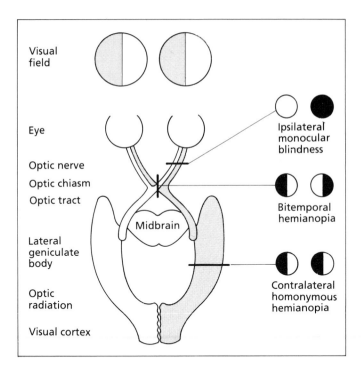

Fig. 12.3. The anatomy of the visual pathways, and the three common types of lesion occurring therein.

improving, the throbbing headache becomes severe. Vasodilatation gives rise to the throbbing headache.

If the vasospasm affects one ophthalmic artery, monocular visual symptoms occur. If the posterior cerebral artery is involved, which is more common, homonymous hemifield visual phenomena occur.

Shimmering, coloured lights, zig-zags, flashing lights are some of the words used to express the positive visual symptoms. Blurring or loss of vision (monocular blindness or homonymous hemianopia) describe the negative visual effects. Complete loss of vision in both eyes is rare in migraine.

Transient ischaemic attacks, infarction, arteritis

Sudden loss of vision of some sort is the characteristic feature. It may be monocular or homonymous hemifield, depending on whether the ophthalmic artery (derived from the internal carotid artery) or the posterior cerebral artery (derived from the vertebro-basilar system) is involved.

Transient ischaemic attacks involving the ophthalmic artery are often described as a curtain coming down over the visual field of one eye, lasting a few minutes, followed by rapid recovery of vision to normal. Very occasionally, embolic material may be seen in the retinal circulation during, or even between, such attacks.

151   *Cranial nerve disorders*

Permanent loss of vision may involve the whole of the visual field of the eye (especially when the posterior ciliary branches of the ophthalmic artery, supplying the optic nerve head regions, are involved). Alternatively, loss of the lower or upper half of one eye's visual field may occur, an altitudinal visual field defect. This indicates selective occlusion of either the upper or lower branch of the central retinal artery in the eye.

The loss of vision in giant cell arteritis is due to arteritic involvement of the posterior ciliary arteries. Loss of vision, in these elderly people, occurs in one eye initially. It is sudden, complete and does not usually recover. Unchecked by steroid treatment, loss of vision in the other eye may follow.

Homonymous hemianopia, due to posterior cerebral artery occlusion, may or may not be noticed by the patient. If central vision is spared, the patient may become aware of the field defect only by bumping into things on the affected side, either with his body, or occasionally with his car! If the homonymous field defect involves central vision on the affected side, the patient usually complains that he can see only half of what he is looking at, which is very noticeable when reading.

Optic neuritis as part of multiple sclerosis

This is described in detail in Chapter 11 (see page 141).

Hereditary, inflammatory, infective or toxic optic neuropathy

Bilateral impairment of visual acuity developing acutely, subacutely or chronically, may be due to a variety of rare diseases affecting the optic nerves. Some examples of such conditions include:

1 acute:
 • methyl alcohol poisoning;
 • bilateral optic neuritis of demyelinating type, usually in children or young people, sometimes as part of Devic's disease (see page 145);
2 subacute:
 • Leber's hereditary optic atrophy;
 • basal meningitis due to sarcoidosis, tuberculosis, malignant infiltration by lymphoma or metastatic cancer;
3 chronic:
 • tobacco/alcohol amblyopia;
 • neurosyphilis.

There may be initial optic disc swelling in acute and subacute cases, but the development of bilateral optic disc pallor is the characteristic finding in these uncommon conditions.

Pituitary and other suprasellar lesions

Bitemporal hemianopia due to optic chiasm compression by a pituitary adenoma growing upwards out of the pituitary fossa is the most classical situation to be considered here (Chapter 7, see page 86). Like most 'classical' syndromes, it is rather unusual in every typical detail because:
• the pituitary tumour does not always grow directly upwards in the midline, so that asymmetrical compression of one optic nerve or one optic tract may occur;
• the precise relationship of pituitary gland and optic chiasm varies from person to person. If the optic chiasm is posteriorly situated, pituitary adenomas are more likely to compress the optic nerves. If the optic chiasm is well forward, optic tract compression is more likely;
• not all suprasellar lesions compressing the optic chiasm are pituitary adenomas. Craniopharyngiomas, meningiomas, and large internal carotid artery aneurysms are alternative, rare, slowly evolving lesions in this vicinity.

Cerebral hemisphere lesions

Though posterior cerebral artery occlusion and infarction of the occipital cortex is the commonest cerebral hemisphere lesion causing permanent visual loss, other hemisphere lesions do cause visual problems:
• an infarct or haematoma in the region of the internal capsule may cause a contralateral homonymous hemianopia, due to involvement of optic tract fibres in the posterior limb of the internal capsule. Contralateral hemiplegia and hemianaesthesia are commonly associated with the visual field defect in patients with lesions in this site;
• vascular lesions, abscesses and tumours situated in the posterior half of the cerebral hemisphere, affecting the optic radiation (between internal capsule and occipital cortex), may cause incomplete or partial homonymous hemianopia. Lesions in the temporal region, affecting the lower parts of the optic radiation, cause homonymous visual field loss in the contralateral upper quadrant. Similarly, by disturbing function in the upper parts of the optic radiation, lesions in the parietal region tend to cause contralateral homonymous lower quadrant field defects. Lesions near, but not physically disrupting, the fibres of the optic radiation may cause

contralateral homonymous visual field neglect. Finger movement may be detected in all parts of the visual field during testing by confrontation of the patient, but bilateral simultaneous visual stimulation by such finger movement may reveal imperfect registration of stimuli from the affected homonymous hemi-field. This is known as visual inattention.

3rd, 4th, and 6th cranial nerves

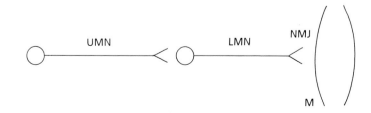

Fig. 12.4. Diagram to show the primary motor pathway.

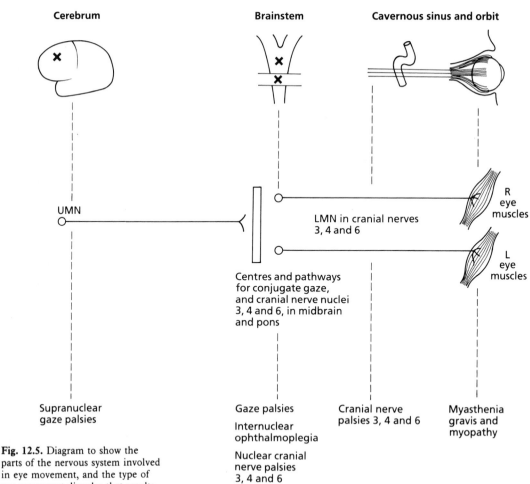

Fig. 12.5. Diagram to show the parts of the nervous system involved in eye movement, and the type of eye movement disorder that results from lesions in each part.

If we recall the primary motor pathway for any voluntary movement (as shown in Fig. 12.4), it becomes apparent that some modification will be necessary in the case of eye movement to enable simultaneous movement of the two eyes, i.e. *conjugate eye movement*. The central part of Fig. 12.5 shows the centres and pathways in the midbrain and pons which act as integrating and coordinating centres, which programme the 3rd, 4th and 6th cranial nerve nuclei to produce conjugate movement of the two eyes. The rest of this section, which is devoted to clinical abnormalities of eye movement, is an elaboration of Fig. 12.5, set out in an annotated and diagrammatic way.

Supranuclear gaze palsy

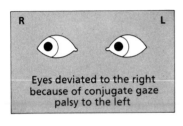

R   L

Eyes deviated to the right because of conjugate gaze palsy to the left

- Site of lesion: cerebral hemisphere.
- Common.
- Common causes:
  massive stroke;
  severe head injury.
- Movement of the eyes to the left is initiated by the right cerebral hemisphere, just like all motor, sensory and visual functions involving the left-hand side of the body. Each cerebral hemisphere has a 'centre' in the frontal region, involved in conjugate deviation of the eyes to the opposite side. Patients with an acute major cerebral hemisphere lesion are unable to deviate their eyes towards the contralateral side. This is the commonest form of supranuclear gaze palsy (right cerebral hemisphere lesion, and paralysis of conjugate gaze to the left in the diagram).
- The centres for conjugate gaze in the brainstem and the cranial nerves are intact. If the brainstem is stimulated reflexly to induce conjugate eye movement, either by caloric stimulation of the ears, or by rapid doll's head movement of the head from side to side, perfectly normal responses will occur. Paralysis of voluntary conjugate gaze, with preserved reflex conjugate eye movement, is the hallmark of supranuclear gaze palsy.

Gaze palsy

At the midbrain level

- Uncommon
- The programming of the 3rd and 4th cranial nerve nuclei for conjugate vertical eye movement, and for convergence of the two eyes, occurs in centres around the aqueduct at superior collicular level. The paralysis of voluntary and

R   L

Eyes won't move up or down in the vertical plane

Eyes won't converge

There may be associated ptosis and pupil abnormality

reflex eye movement which occurs with lesions in this region is known as Parinaud's syndrome.

At the pontine level

- Uncommon
- Conjugation of the two eyes in horizontal eye movements is achieved by an ipsilateral pontine gaze centre, as shown in Fig. 12.6. A lesion in the lateral pontine region (on the right in the diagram) will cause voluntary and reflex paralysis of conjugate gaze towards the side of the lesion.

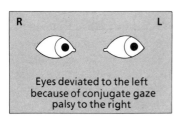

Eyes deviated to the left because of conjugate gaze palsy to the right

Fig. 12.6. Brainstem centres and pathways for conjugate horizontal movement. Voluntary gaze to the left is initiated in the right cerebral hemisphere. A descending pathway from the right cerebral hemisphere innervates the left pontine gaze centre. From there, impulses pass directly to the left 6th nerve nucleus to abduct the left eye, and (via the medial longitudinal fasciculus) to the right 3rd nerve nucleus to adduct the right eye.

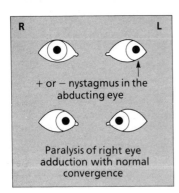

+ or − nystagmus in the abducting eye

Paralysis of right eye adduction with normal convergence

Internuclear ophthalmoplegia

- Site of lesion: midbrain/pons (see Fig. 12.6).
- Common.
- Common cause: multiple sclerosis.

A lesion between the 3rd nerve nucleus in the midbrain and the 6th nerve nucleus in the pons — an internuclear lesion — on the course of the medial longitudinal fasciculus (on the right side in the diagram):

156 *Chapter 12*

- does not interfere with activation of the left 6th nerve nucleus in the pons from the left pontine gaze centre, so that abduction of the left eye is normal (except for some nystagmus which is difficult to explain);
- does interfere with activation of the right 3rd nerve nucleus in the midbrain from the left pontine gaze centre, so that adduction of the right eye may be slow, incomplete or paralysed;
- does not interfere with activation of either 3rd nerve nucleus by the midbrain convergence coordinating centres, so that convergence of the eyes is normal.

Before considering 3rd, 4th and 6th nerve palsies in detail, it is worth remembering the individual action of each of the eye muscles, and their innervation (Fig. 12.7).

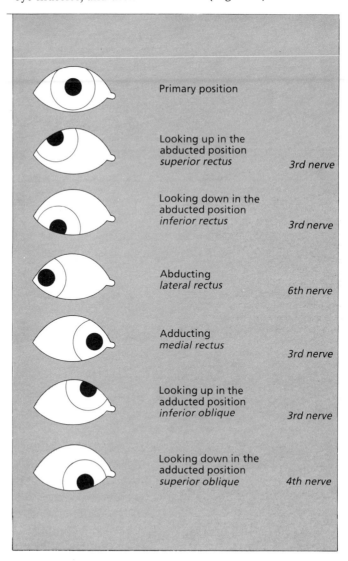

Primary position

Looking up in the abducted position
superior rectus   *3rd nerve*

Looking down in the abducted position
inferior rectus   *3rd nerve*

Abducting
lateral rectus   *6th nerve*

Adducting
medial rectus   *3rd nerve*

Looking up in the adducted position
inferior oblique   *3rd nerve*

Looking down in the adducted position
superior oblique   *4th nerve*

Fig. 12.7. Normal eye movements in terms of which muscle and which nerve effect them. Diagram shows the right eye viewed from the front.

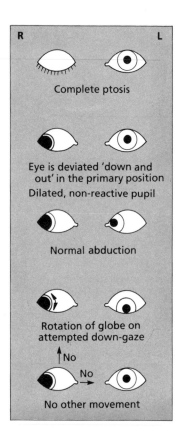

R   L

Complete ptosis

Eye is deviated 'down and out' in the primary position
Dilated, non-reactive pupil

Normal abduction

Rotation of globe on attempted down-gaze

↑No

No →

No other movement

3rd nerve palsy

- Common.
- Common causes:
  posterior communicating artery aneurysm (painful);
  mononeuritis in diabetes (pupil usually normal);
  pathology beside the cavernous sinus, in the superior orbital fissure or in the orbit (adjacent nerves commonly involved, e.g. 4, 6, 5a, and 2 if in the orbit).
- The parasympathetic innervation of the eye is supplied by the 3rd nerve.
- The diagram shows a complete right 3rd nerve palsy. The lesion can be incomplete of course, in terms of ptosis, pupil dilatation, or weakness of eye movement.

4th nerve palsy

- Uncommon.
- Common cause: trauma affecting the orbit.

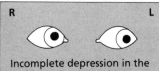

R   L

Incomplete depression in the adducted position (right eye in this diagram)

Some torsion of the eye in the orbit

Compensatory head tilt towards the opposite shoulder may be present, to obtain single vision whilst looking forward

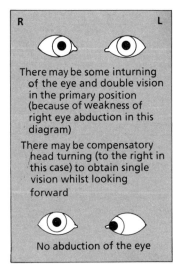

R   L

There may be some inturning of the eye and double vision in the primary position (because of weakness of right eye abduction in this diagram)

There may be compensatory head turning (to the right in this case) to obtain single vision whilst looking forward

No abduction of the eye

6th nerve palsy

- Common.
- Common causes:
  as a false localizing sign in patients with raised intracranial pressure;
  multiple sclerosis and small cerebrovascular lesions within the pons;
  pathology beside the cavernous sinus, in the superior orbital fissure or orbit (adjacent nerves commonly involved, e.g. 3, 4, 5a, and 2 if in the orbit).

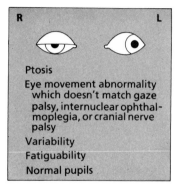

Ptosis

Eye movement abnormality which doesn't match gaze palsy, internuclear ophthalmoplegia, or cranial nerve palsy

Variability

Fatiguability

Normal pupils

Myasthenia gravis

- Uncommon.
- Ocular involvement common in myasthenia gravis.
- Myasthenia should be considered in any unexplained ophthalmoplegia, even if it looks like a 6th or partial 3rd nerve palsy.

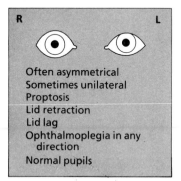

Often asymmetrical

Sometimes unilateral

Proptosis

Lid retraction

Lid lag

Ophthalmoplegia in any direction

Normal pupils

Myopathy

- Graves' disease is the only common myopathy to involve eye muscles.
- The patient may be hyperthyroid, euthyroid, or hypothyroid.
- Inflammatory swelling of the external ocular muscles and fat within the orbit, often leading to fibrosis, is responsible.
- Involvement of the external ocular muscles in other forms of myopathy occurs, but is exceedingly rare.

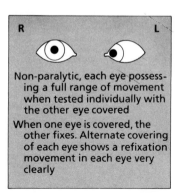

Non-paralytic, each eye possessing a full range of movement when tested individually with the other eye covered

When one eye is covered, the other fixes. Alternate covering of each eye shows a refixation movement in each eye very clearly

Concomitant squint

- Very common.
- Caused by dissimilar visual acuity and refractive properties in the two eyes from an early age.
- Proper binocular fixation has never been established.
- Known as amblyopia.
- Fixation is by the better seeing eye, the image from the amblyopic eye is suppressed, so there is no complaint of double vision.

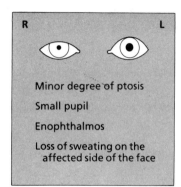

Minor degree of ptosis

Small pupil

Enophthalmos

Loss of sweating on the affected side of the face

Horner's syndrome

- Uncommon.
- Caused by loss of sympathetic innervation to the eye.
- The sympathetic supply to the face and eye is derived from the hypothalamic region, descends ipsilaterally through the brainstem and cervical cord, and reaches the sympathetic chain via the motor root of T1. From the superior cervical sympathetic ganglion, the fibres pass along the outer sheath of the common carotid artery. Fibres to the eye travel via the internal carotid artery and its ophthalmic branch. Fibres to the face travel with the external carotid artery and its branches.

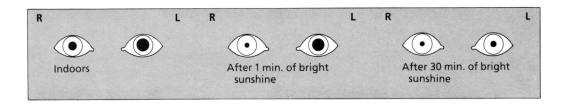

R	L	R	L	R	L
Indoors		After 1 min. of bright sunshine		After 30 min. of bright sunshine	

Holmes–Adie syndrome (illustrated above)

- Uncommon.
- Often unilateral.
- An interesting curiosity of no sinister significance.
- Very slow pupillary reaction to light and accommodation (left eye in diagram).
- Absent deep tendon reflexes in the limbs is a common accompaniment, especially knee and ankle jerks.
- Site of pathology uncertain.

Argyll–Robertson pupil

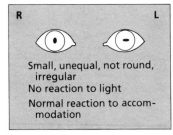

R   L

Small, unequal, not round, irregular
No reaction to light
Normal reaction to accommodation

- Uncommon.
- A sign of tertiary syphilis.
- Site of pathology uncertain (?peri-aqueductal region of the midbrain).

Orbital mass lesions

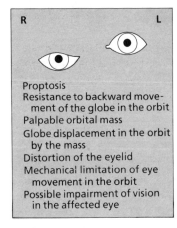

R   L

Proptosis
Resistance to backward movement of the globe in the orbit
Palpable orbital mass
Globe displacement in the orbit by the mass
Distortion of the eyelid
Mechanical limitation of eye movement in the orbit
Possible impairment of vision in the affected eye

- Uncommon.
- Causes:
  benign tumours;
  malignant tumours, primary or secondary;
  extension of inflammatory pathology from the paranasal sinuses;
  non-neoplastic inflammatory infiltrate at the back of the orbit, so-called 'pseudotumour'.
- CT scanning of the orbits is the most helpful investigation.

Trigeminal nerve

Sensory loss in the face is very noticeable, as a visit to the dentist which requires a local anaesthetic will remind us. Sensory loss affecting the cornea can lead unwittingly to serious corneal damage. Pain in the face is very intrusive.

Figures 12.8 and 12.9 demonstrate the relevant clinical anatomical features of the trigeminal nerve. The following points are worth noting:
- the upper border of sensory loss in a trigeminal nerve lesion lies between the ear and the vertex, and the lower

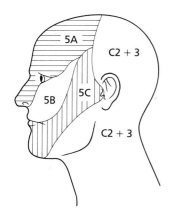

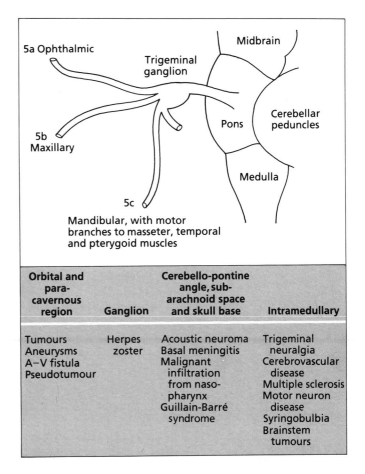

Orbital and para-cavernous region	Ganglion	Cerebello-pontine angle, sub-arachnoid space and skull base	Intramedullary
Tumours Aneurysms A–V fistula Pseudotumour	Herpes zoster	Acoustic neuroma Basal meningitis Malignant infiltration from naso-pharynx Guillain-Barré syndrome	Trigeminal neuralgia Cerebrovascular disease Multiple sclerosis Motor neuron disease Syringobulbia Brainstem tumours

Fig. 12.9. (*right*) Diagram to show the trigeminal nerve, and the diseases that may affect it.

border is above the angle of the jaw. Patients who are affecting sensory loss on the face tend to have the junction of forehead and scalp as the upper border, and the angle of the jaw as the lower border;

• the corneal reflex requires corneal, not scleral, stimulation, and the response (mediated through the 7th cranial nerve) is to blink bilaterally. It can therefore be tested in the presence of an ipsilateral 7th nerve lesion;

• the jaw-jerk, like any other stretch reflex, is exaggerated in the presence of an upper motor neurone lesion. In the case of the jaw-jerk, the lesion must be above the level of the trigeminal motor nucleus in the pons. In patients with upper motor neurone signs in all four limbs, an exaggerated jaw-jerk is sometimes helpful in suggesting that the lesion is above the pons, rather than between the pons and the mid-cervical region of the spinal cord;

• paracavernous pathology affects only the ophthalmic and maxillary branches of the trigeminal nerve, as the mandibular branch has dived through the foramen ovale, behind the cavernous sinus. Similarly, orbital pathology affects only the ophthalmic branch, since the maxillary branch has exited

161 *Cranial nerve disorders*

the skull through the foramen rotundum posterior to the orbit.

Figure 12.9 gives information about the diseases that may affect the trigeminal nerve. There are really only two common ones: trigeminal neuralgia and Herpes zoster.

• *Trigeminal neuralgia* is described in Chapter 3 (see page 40), and must be the most common disease affecting the trigeminal nerve. Though included in the intramedullary column of the table in the lower half of Fig. 12.9, the precise nature and location of the lesion in this condition remains uncertain. Some form of abnormal paroxysmal electrical discharge in the sensory nucleus of the trigeminal nerve is the rather vague notion associated with trigeminal neuralgia.

• *Herpes zoster* (shingles) affecting the trigeminal nerve is also mentioned in Chapter 3 (see page 41) and in Chapter 16 (page 223). Though the virus is in the trigeminal ganglion, clinical involvement is most usually confined to the skin and cornea supplied by the ophthalmic branch. The painful vesicular rash, sometimes preceded by pain for a few days and sometimes followed by pain for ever, is similar to shingles elsewhere in the body. The involvement of the cornea, however, makes urgent ophthalmic referral essential, and the use of local, oral, or parenteral antiviral agents (like acyclovir) important. Parenteral administration is especially likely if there is any evidence of immuno-suppression in the patient.

Facial nerve

Figure 12.10 shows the peripheral distribution of the facial nerve. The nerve leaves the pons in the cerebello-pontine angle. It provides autonomic efferent fibres to lacrimal and salivary glands, collects afferent taste fibres from the anterior two-thirds of the tongue, and provides the innervation of the stapedius muscle in the ear, before emerging from the stylomastoid foramen behind and below the ear to innervate the facial muscles as shown in Fig. 12.10.

Proximal lesions of the facial nerve produce therefore, in addition to weakness of all the ipsilateral facial muscles, an alteration of secretion in the ipsilateral lacrimal and salivary glands, impairment of taste perception on the anterior two-thirds of the tongue, and hyperacusis (sounds heard abnormally loudly) in the ear on the side of the lesion. If the lesion has been complete, with Wallerian axonal degeneration distal to the site of the lesion, recovery is rarely complete and re-innervation is often incorrect. Axons, which used to supply the lower part of the face, may re-grow along

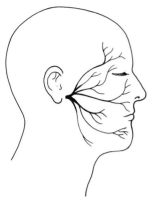

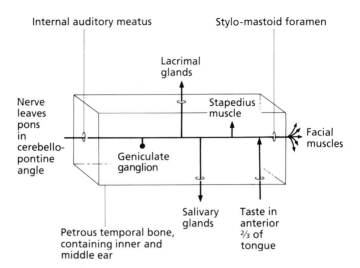

Internal auditory meatus   Stylo-mastoid foramen

Lacrimal glands

Nerve leaves pons in cerebello-pontine angle

Stapedius muscle

Geniculate ganglion

Facial muscles

Salivary glands   Taste in anterior ⅔ of tongue

Petrous temporal bone, containing inner and middle ear

Fig. 12.10. The peripheral distribution of the facial nerve to the muscles of the face, and a highly diagrammatic representation of the proximal part of the facial nerve within the petrous temporal bone.

Schwann tubes which lead to the upper part of the face, and vice versa. Patients in whom this has happened are unable to contract part of their facial muscles in isolation. When they close their eyes vigorously, there is retraction of the corner of the mouth on the affected side. When they contract mouth muscles as in whistling, there is eye muscle contraction and possible closure on the side of the lesion. Sometimes, axons that used to supply the salivary glands find their way to the lacrimal glands. In such patients, tears may form excessively in the eye of the affected side at mealtimes.

Bell's palsy

The common disease of the facial nerve is Bell's palsy. The cause of this condition, and the precise site of pathology, are not certain, though the lesion is usually proximal enough to have effects on taste and hearing. After some aching in the region of the ear, the facial weakness develops quite quickly within 24 hours. The patient is usually very concerned by the facial appearance. Drainage of tears from the eye may be disturbed on the affected side because the eyelids lose close apposition with the globe of the eye, so the eye waters. The cornea may be vulnerable because of impaired eye closure. Speaking, eating, and drinking may be difficult because of the weakness around the mouth.

If the facial palsy is not complete, and if the facial nerve remains excitable on electrical stimulation below the ear, then recovery usually occurs in weeks and is complete. This is because the damage has been confined to the myelin sheaths without axonal damage. If the palsy is complete and the nerve becomes inexcitable after a few days, then Wallerian degeneration has probably occurred distal to the

163   *Cranial nerve disorders*

site of the lesion. Recovery will be slow, disappointing, incomplete, and incorrect.

Care of the eye, encouragement, facial exercises in the mirror are all that can be offered in the way of treatment in the acute stage, unless the patient is seen within 12–24 hours of onset when a short course of steroids may improve the patient's prospects for recovery.

Plastic surgery, or facio-hypoglossal nerve anastomosis, may be offered later if recovery has been very disappointing. (In the latter procedure, the ipsilateral hypoglossal nerve is divided and the proximal part is anastomosed to the non-functional facial nerve. Axonal growth along the facial nerve may improve tone and movement in the facial muscles to give the patient some satisfaction.)

Rarer causes of facial palsy

- *Herpes zoster* affecting the geniculate ganglion, which lies on the course of the facial nerve. Vesicles may appear in the external auditory meatus or soft palate to indicate this cause of the facial palsy. This is known as the Ramsay–Hunt syndrome and behaves like an idiopathic Bell's palsy from the point of view of recovery;
- *Trauma*, fractures involving the petrous temporal bone;
- *Middle ear infection*, acute or chronic;
- *Diabetes mellitus;*
- *Sarcoidosis;*
- *Acoustic neuroma*, either before or after its removal from the cerebello-pontine angle;
- *Surgery* in the ear and parotid gland region;
- *Lyme disease.*

There is an uncommon but embarrassing conditon of the facial nerve known as *clonic hemifacial spasm*, in which there is intermittent spontaneous contraction of the facial muscles on one side of the face. There is sometimes evidence of a partial lower motor neurone facial weakness. The condition is a great embarrassment, difficult to treat, and rarely symptomatic of any serious condition of the facial nerve.

Cochleo-vestibular nerve

Figure 12.11 reminds us of the extremely delicate structure of the cochlea and labyrinth within the petrous temporal bone, of the radiation of incoming information from the inner ear throughout the CNS, and of the localization of auditory and vestibular functions in the posterior part of the superior temporal gyrus in the cerebral hemisphere.

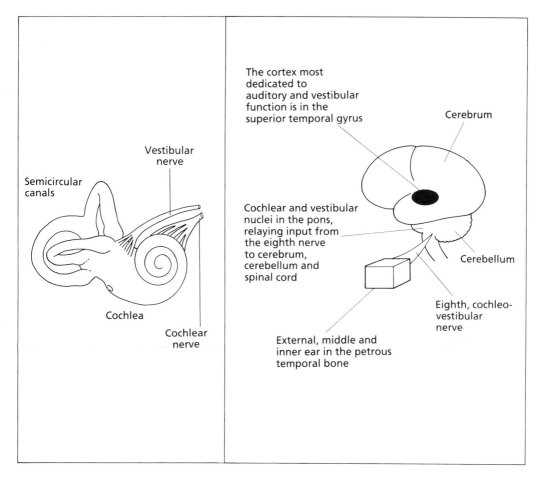

Fig. 12.11. The left-hand side of the diagram shows detail of the inner ear in the petrous temporal bone. The right-hand side of the diagram shows the central connections of the 8th nerve.

Main symptoms of cochleo-vestibular disease

These are:
- *deafness*, on one or both sides;
- *tinnitus*, all sorts of different noises heard in one or both ears or in the head;
- *vertigo*, a sensation of movement of the environment with respect to the patient;
- *loss of balance*, affecting walking, standing or even sitting in extreme cases.

Abnormal physical signs in cochleo-vestibular disease

The particular abnormal physical signs to be sought in patients with these symptoms are as follows.

Deafness

If the patient is unable to hear the whispered voice in one or both ears, a check should be made to find out whether the

165 *Cranial nerve disorders*

deafness is conductive (external or middle ear) or nerve (perceptive) deafness. This is done by Rinne's test. If bone conduction is better than air conduction, i.e. there is conductive deafness, a lesion in the external or middle ear should be sought. Otoscopic examination of the external auditory canal (for wax) and eardrum should be the next thing to do. If air conduction is better than bone conduction, a lesion of the cochlea or 8th nerve should be pursued.

Nystagmus

Patients with lesions in the labyrinth, 8th nerve, vestibular nucleus and its central connections in the CNS frequently show nystagmus, which is more evident on eye deviation towards the side of the lesion.

Ataxia

Patients with vertigo and nystagmus due to labyrinthine disease, 8th nerve or brainstem lesions may all show gait ataxia, with falling towards the side of the lesion. Other cerebellar signs (dysarthria, limb ataxia in finger–nose and heel–knee–shin testing) strongly indicate that the lesion is central, rather than in the labyrinth.

Positional nystagmus

Some patients complaining of vertigo have no nystagmus at rest during normal neurological examination, but exhibit vertigo and nystagmus after a sudden change in position of the head. From the seated position on the examination couch, the patient is asked to lie down rapidly on his back, with the head being held by the examiner in a position of rotation to either side. Nystagmus, which is induced after a short delay, associated with extreme vertigo, which fatigues after a few seconds, and which becomes more difficult to elicit on the second and the third testing, indicates the presence of the labyrinthine disorder known as benign paroxysmal positional vertigo. Nystagmus which is induced in this way in more than one position, with little vertigo and little diminution on successive testing, is more characteristic of brainstem lesions.

Common tests for cochleo-vestibular disease

The common tests which are used to help to elucidate the nature of cochleo-vestibular complaints are:

Audiometry

In which hearing at different sound frequencies is plotted for each ear.

Various evoked potential recording techniques

In which responses in the ear and from the scalp near the ear, are recorded (using repetitive stimulation and summation of responses by an averaging computer). Characteristic defects in the wave form of the evoked response occur with lesions at different sites, e.g. cochlea, auditory nerve, brainstem.

Caloric tests

Stimulation of the labyrinth by irrigation of the external auditory canals by hot and cold water produces nystagmus in the primary position in normal people. Loss or asymmetry of response to such stimulation may be found in peripheral labyrinthine or central brainstem lesions.

Electronystagmography

Movements of the eyes can be recorded by electrodes applied to each side of the eye. The output from such electrodes can be used to form a permanent record of nystagmus in the primary position during fixation of the eyes, in the dark (no fixation), on eye deviation to one or other side, during caloric stimulation, and during optokinetic stimulation when the patient's eyes are looking at a striped revolving drum. Features of the nystagmus recorded in this way can help to localize the site of a vestibular lesion.

Common causes of deafness and loss of balance

Figure 12.12 demonstrates that the common causes of deafness are in the external, middle or inner ear. *Acoustic neuroma* is an occasional cause of slowly progressive unilateral nerve deafness. Ideally, it should be diagnosed and treated at this stage, before it has caused other evidence of a cerebello-pontine space-occupying lesion (i.e. 5th and 7th cranial nerve palsy, ipsilateral cerebellar signs, and raised intracranial pressure by distorting the 4th ventricle and interfering with the flow of CSF through it). The tumour is a benign one, derived from the Schwann cells on the 8th nerve, so it is tragic to allow it to become too large for safe and complete removal.

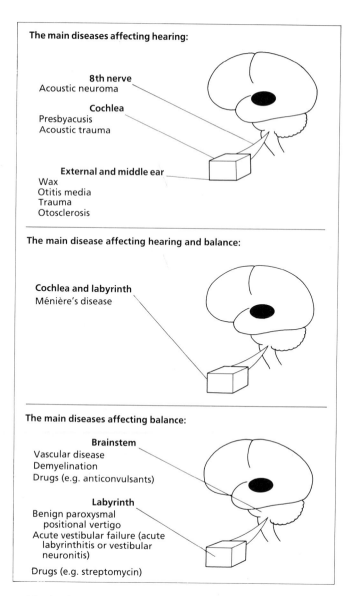

The main diseases affecting hearing:

8th nerve
Acoustic neuroma

Cochlea
Presbyacusis
Acoustic trauma

External and middle ear
Wax
Otitis media
Trauma
Otosclerosis

The main disease affecting hearing and balance:

Cochlea and labyrinth
Ménière's disease

The main diseases affecting balance:

Brainstem
Vascular disease
Demyelination
Drugs (e.g. anticonvulsants)

Labyrinth
Benign paroxysmal
  positional vertigo
Acute vestibular failure (acute
  labyrinthitis or vestibular
  neuronitis)
Drugs (e.g. streptomycin)

Fig. 12.12. The main diseases affecting hearing, balance, or both .

Ménière's disease is depicted in the central section of Fig. 12.12. It is probably due to a lesion in the endolymph in both the cochlea and the labyrinth. It therefore causes auditory and vestibular symptoms. A middle-aged person with a history of unilateral deafness and tinnitus, who becomes subject to episodes of very severe vertigo, vomiting, and ataxia lasting a few hours, constitutes the typical clinical picture of this condition. It is not easy to treat.

The common diseases to affect balance without hearing loss are shown in the lower part of Fig. 12.12. It can be seen that the lesion is likely to be central in the brainstem, or peripheral in the labyrinth.

Episodes of *ischaemia* or *infarction* in the brainstem, or episodes of *demyelination* in patients with multiple sclerosis, are the common structural lesions in the brainstem to disturb balance. Such lesions commonly produce other neurological signs (cranial nerve, cerebellar or long tract in the limbs).

The clues to the diagnosis of *benign paroxysmal positional vertigo* are:
• intermittent transient vertigo lasting less than 30 seconds strongly related to putting the head into a specific position. Turning over in bed, lying down in bed, and looking upwards, are common precipitants;
• perfect health otherwise;
• no abnormalities on routine examination;
• definite positional nystagmus with the characteristics described earlier in this section;
• spontaneous resolution of the problem after a few months.

Perhaps the commonest type of severe vertigo is due to *sudden vestibular failure*. This denotes the sudden occurrence of rotatory vertigo, gait ataxia, vomiting, and the need to stay in bed. Lateralized nystagmus and gait ataxia are the two abnormal physical signs. The incapacity lasts very severely for a few days and then gradually resolves over 4–6 weeks. Head movement aggravates the symptoms so the patient keeps still in bed in the acute stage, and walks with his head rather set on his shoulders in the convalescent stage.

The underlying pathology is not certain. The problem may follow an upper respiratory infection and occasionally occurs in epidemics, hence the use of the diagnostic terms *acute labyrinthitis* or *vestibular neuronitis*. In the elderly, it may be the consequence of occlusive vascular disease affecting the labyrinth.

Three last points in this section:
1 Though auditory and vestibular phenomena occasionally feature in *temporal lobe epilepsy*, cerebral hemisphere lesions rarely cause cochleo-vestibular symptoms.
2 Drugs that impair balance include:
   • amino-glycoside antibiotics, such as streptomycin and gentamicin, which may permanently impair vestibular function if toxic blood levels are allowed to accumulate;
   • anticonvulsants, barbiturates, and alcohol which impair the function of the brainstem/cerebellum whilst blood levels are too high.
3 Drugs that relieve or diminish vertigo include:
   • cinnarizine;
   • prochlorperazine;
   • betahistine.

Glossopharyngeal, vagus, and hypoglossal nerves

These three lower cranial nerves are considered in one section of this chapter for two reasons.

1 Together they innervate the mouth and throat for normal speech and swallowing.

2 They are commonly involved in disease processes together, to give rise to the clinical picture of bulbar palsy.

More specifically, the glossopharyngeal nerve supplies the palate and pharynx, the vagus nerve supplies the pharynx and larynx, and the hypoglossal nerve supplies the tongue. Taste perception in the posterior third of the tongue is a function of the glossopharyngeal nerve. Both the glossopharyngeal and vagus nerves (especially the latter) have an enormous autonomic function, as shown in Fig. 12.13. Innervation of the vocal cords by the long, thin, recurrent laryngeal nerves (from the vagus) exposes them to possible damage as far down as the subclavian artery on the right, and the arch of the aorta on the left.

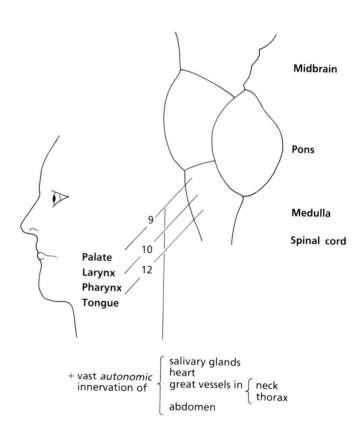

Fig. 12.13. Highly diagrammatic representation of cranial nerves 9, 10, and 12.

Bulbar palsy

When there is bilateral impairment of function in the 9th, 10th, and 12th cranial nerves, the clinical syndrome of bulbar palsy evolves. The features of bulbar palsy are:
- *dysarthria;*
- *dysphagia,* often with choking episodes and/or nasal regurgitation of fluids;
- *dysphonia* and *poor cough,* because of weak vocal cords;
- *susceptibility to aspiration pneumonia.*

Even though the vagus nerve has a vast and important autonomic role, it is uncommon for autonomic abnormalities to feature in the diseases discussed in this section.

Common conditions affecting 9th, 10th, and 12th nerve function

Figure 12.14 illustrates the common conditions which affect 9th, 10th, and 12th nerve function. The use of the word common is relative, since none of the conditions is very common.

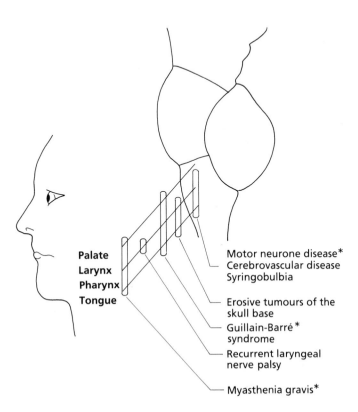

Palate
Larynx
Pharynx
Tongue

Motor neurone disease*
Cerebrovascular disease
Syringobulbia

Erosive tumours of the skull base

Guillain-Barré* syndrome

Recurrent laryngeal nerve palsy

Myasthenia gravis*

Fig. 12.14. Common conditions that affect cranial nerves 9,10, and 12. * Because these conditions involve 9th, 10th and 12th nerve function bilaterally, they are the common causes of bulbar palsy.

Motor neurone disease

When motor neurone disease is causing loss of motor neurones from the lower cranial motor nuclei in the medulla, the bulbar palsy can eventually lead to extreme difficulty in speech (anarthria) and swallowing. Inanition and aspiration pneumonia are commonly responsible for such patients' deaths. The tongue is small, weak or immobile, and fasciculating (Chapter 14, see page 190).

Infarction of the lateral medulla

Infarction of the lateral medulla, following posterior inferior cerebellar artery occlusion, is one of the most dramatic cerebrovascular syndromes to involve speech and swallowing. (A major neurological deficit results from a small area of infarction in a part of the brain containing many important nuclei and fibre pathways.) Ipsilateral trigeminal, vestibular, glossopharyngeal, and vagal nuclei may be involved, along with cerebellar and spino-thalamic fibre tracts in the lateral medulla.

Guillain-Barré syndrome

Patients with Guillain–Barré syndrome, acute, post-infectious polyneuropathy (Chapter 14, see page 196), may need ventilation via an endotracheal tube or cuffed tracheotomy tube. This may be necessary either because of neuropathic weakness of the chest wall and diaphragm, or because of bulbar palsy secondary to lower cranial nerve involvement in the neuropathy.

Recurrent laryngeal nerve palsy

The recurrent laryngeal nerves are vulnerable to damage in the neck and mediastinum, e.g. aortic aneurysm, malignant chest tumours, malignant glands and surgery in the neck (especially in the region of the thyroid gland). A unilateral vocal cord palsy due to a unilateral nerve lesion produces little disability other than slight hoarseness. Bilateral vocal cord paralysis is much more disabling, with marked hoarseness of the voice, a weak 'bovine' cough (because the cords cannot be strongly adducted), and respiratory stridor.

Myasthenia gravis

Bulbar muscle involvement in myasthenia gravis is quite common in this rare condition. The fatiguability of muscle function, which characterizes this condition, is frequently very noticeable in the patient's speech and swallowing.

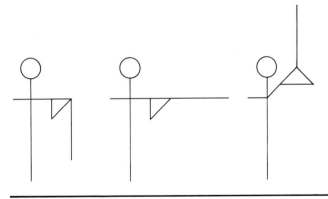

Fig. 12.15. The importance of the trapezius muscle in arm elevation.

The first half of the shoulder abduction requires good scapula stabilization by trapezius (and other muscles), so that deltoid muscle contraction can take the arm to the horizontal position.

The second half of the shoulder abduction requires elevation of the shoulder and scapula rotation through almost 90° by trapezius (and other muscles).

The spinal accessory nerve

This nerve arises from the upper segments of the cervical spinal cord, ascends into the skull through the foramen magnum, only to exit the skull again with the 9th and 10th cranial nerves through the jugular foramen. The nerve then travels down the side of the neck to supply the sternomastoid muscle, and then crosses the posterior triangle of the neck quite superficially to supply the upper parts of the trapezius muscle.

Lesions of this nerve are uncommon. It is very vulnerable to surgical trauma in the posterior triangle of the neck. Loss of function in the upper part of the trapezius muscle produces a significant disability in the shoulder region. The scapula and shoulder sag downwards and outwards in the resting position. Arm elevation is impaired because of poor scapular stability and rotation, as illustrated in Fig. 12.15.

Chapter 13

Nerve root, nerve plexus and peripheral nerve lesions

Introduction

In this chapter, we are considering focal pathology in the peripheral nervous system. This means a study of the effect of lesions between the spinal cord and the distal connections of the peripheral nerves with skin, joints and muscles (as shown in Fig. 13.1). We shall become familiar with focal disease affecting nerve roots and spinal nerves, nerve plexuses and individual peripheral nerves. Focal disease infers a single localized lesion, affecting one nerve root or one peripheral nerve. Diffuse or generalized diseases affecting these parts of the nervous system, e.g. a peripheral neuropathy affecting all the peripheral nerves throughout the body, are the subject of Chapter 14.

Focal lesions of the lower cervical and lower lumbar nerve roots are common, as are certain individual peripheral nerve lesions in the limbs. Accurate recognition of these clinical syndromes depends on some basic neuro-anatomical knowledge. This is not formidably complicated but possession of a few hard anatomical facts is inescapable.

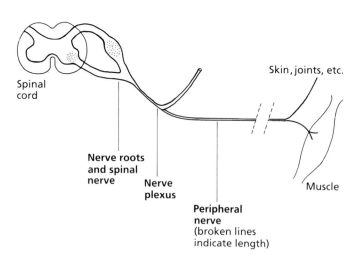

Fig. 13.1. Schematic diagram of the peripheral nervous system.

Nerve root lesions

Figure 13.2 is a representation of the position of the nerve roots and spinal nerve in relation to skeletal structures. The precise position of the union of the ventral and dorsal nerve roots, to form the spinal nerve, in the intervertebral foramen is a little variable. This is why a consideration of the clinical problems affecting nerve roots embraces those affecting the spinal nerve. A nerve root lesion, radiculopathy, suggests a

Fig. 13.2. Superior aspect of a cervical vertebra, and lateral aspect of the lumbar spine.

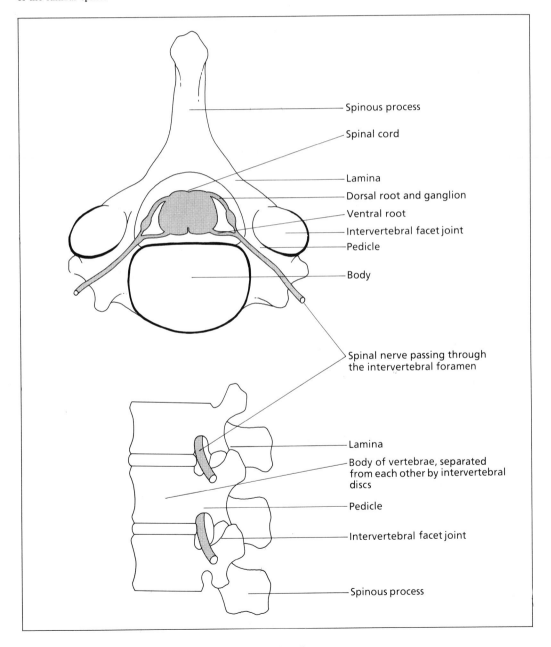

Spinous process

Spinal cord

Lamina
Dorsal root and ganglion
Ventral root
Intervertebral facet joint
Pedicle

Body

Spinal nerve passing through the intervertebral foramen

Lamina
Body of vertebrae, separated from each other by intervertebral discs

Pedicle

Intervertebral facet joint

Spinous process

lesion involving the dorsal and ventral nerve roots and/or the spinal nerve.

The common syndromes associated with pathology of the nerve roots and spinal nerves are:

- *prolapsed intervertebral disc;*
- *Herpes zoster;*
- *metastatic disease in the spine.*

Less common is the compression of these structures by a *neurofibroma.*

Prolapsed intervertebral disc

When the central, softer material, nucleus pulposus, of an intervertebral disc protrudes through a tear in the outer skin, anulus fibrosus, the situation is known as a prolapsed intervertebral disc. This is by far the most common pathology to affect nerve roots and spinal nerves. The susceptibility of these nerve elements to disc prolapses, which are most commonly postero-lateral in or near the intervertebral foramen, is well shown in Fig. 13.2.

The typical clinical features of a prolapsed intervertebral disc, regardless of the level, are:

1 *Skeletal*
- pain, tenderness, and limitation in the range of movement in the affected area of the spine;
- reduced straight leg raising on the side of the lesion, in the case of lumbar disc prolapses.

2 *Neurological*
- pain, sensory symptoms, and sensory loss in the dermatome of the affected nerve root;
- lower motor neurone signs (weakness and wasting) in the myotome of the affected nerve root;
- loss of tendon reflexes of the appropriate segmental value;
- since most disc prolapses are postero-lateral, these neurological features are almost always unilateral.

Prolapsed intervertebral discs are most common between C4 and T1 in the cervical spine and between L3 and S1 in the lumbo-sacral spine. In the cervical region, there is not a great discrepancy between the level of the cervical spinal cord segment and the cervical vertebra of the same number, i.e. the C5 segment of spinal cord, the C5 nerve roots and the C4/5 intervertebral foramen, through which the C5 spinal nerve passes, are all at much the same level (see Fig. 10.1). If the patient presents with a C5 neurological deficit therefore, it is very likely that it will be a C4/5 intervertebral disc prolapse.

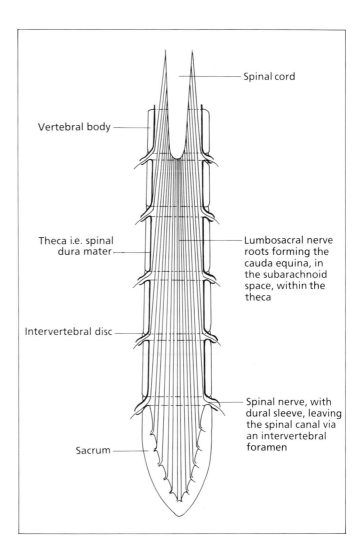

Spinal cord

Vertebral body

Theca i.e. spinal
dura mater

Lumbosacral nerve
roots forming the
cauda equina, in
the subarachnoid
space, within the
theca

Intervertebral disc

Spinal nerve, with
dural sleeve, leaving
the spinal canal via
an intervertebral
foramen

Sacrum

Fig. 13.3. Posterior view of the
cauda equina. *NB* The pedicles,
laminae, and spinous processes of
the vertebrae, and the posterior half
of the theca, have been removed.

Figures 10.1 and 13.3 show that this is not the case in the
lumbar region. The lower end of the spinal cord is at the
level of the L1 vertebra. All the lumbar and sacral nerve
roots have to descend over a considerable length to reach the
particular intervertebral foramen through which they exit
the spinal canal. These nerve roots form the cauda equina,
lying within the theca. Each nerve root passes laterally,
within a sheath of dura, at the level at which it passes
through the intervertebral foramen. Postero-lateral disc
prolapses are likely to compress the emerging spinal nerve
within the intervertebral foramen, e.g. an L4/5 disc prolapse
will compress the emerging L4 root. More medially situated
disc prolapses in the lumbar region may compress nerve
roots of lower numerical value, which are going to exit the
spinal canal lower down. This is more likely to happen if the
patient has a constitutionally narrow spinal canal. (Some

177 *Peripheral nervous system*

individuals have wide capacious spinal canals, others have short stubby pedicles and laminae to give a small cross-sectional area for the cauda equina.) It cannot be assumed therefore that an L5 root syndrome is the consequence of an L5/S1 disc prolapse; the trouble may be higher up. A more centrally prolapsed lumbar disc may produce bilateral leg symptoms and signs, involving more than one segment, often associated with sphincter malfunction due to lower sacral nerve root compression.

Figures 13.4 and 13.5 show the segmental value of the movements, reflexes, and skin sensation most frequently involved in cervical and lumbar disc disease. From these diagrams, the area of pain and sensory malfunction, the location of weakness and wasting, and the impaired deep tendon reflexes can all be identified for any single nerve root syndrome. (Note that Figs 13.4 and 13.5 indicate weak movements, not the actual site of the weak and wasted muscles, which are of course proximal to the joints being moved.)

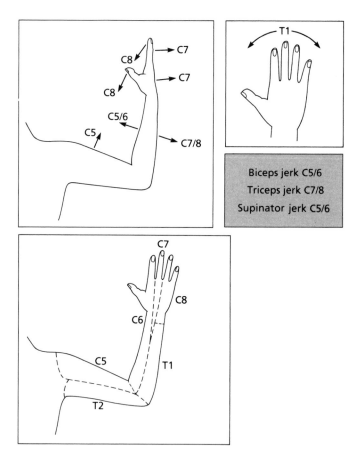

Biceps jerk C5/6
Triceps jerk C7/8
Supinator jerk C5/6

Fig. 13.4. Segmental nerve supply to the upper limb, in terms of movements, tendon reflexes, and skin sensation.

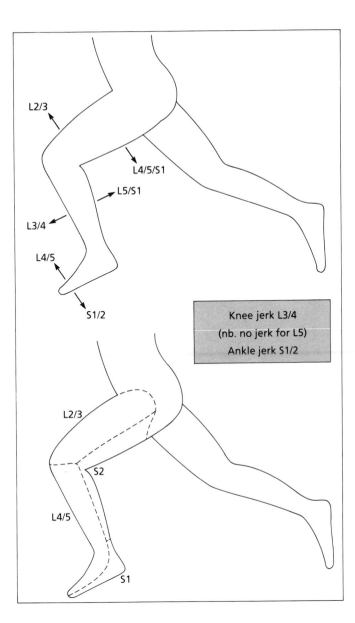

Fig. 13.5. Segmental nerve supply to the lower limb, in terms of movements, tendon reflexes, and skin sensation.

Labels in figure:
L2/3
L4/5/S1
L5/S1
L3/4
L4/5
S1/2

Knee jerk L3/4
(nb. no jerk for L5)
Ankle jerk S1/2

L2/3
S2
L4/5
S1

There are four main intervertebral disc disease syndromes.

1 The single, acute disc prolapse which is sudden, often related to unusually heavy lifting or exertion, very incapacitating, often associated with symptoms and signs of nerve root compression, and requiring bed rest, whether it affects the cervical or lumbar region.

2 More gradually evolving, multiple level disc herniation in association with osteo-arthritis of the spine. Disc degeneration is associated with osteophyte formation, not just in the main intervertebral joint between body and body, but also in the interfacet joints. Figure 13.2 shows how osteo-arthritic

179 *Peripheral nervous system*

changes in the interfacet joint may further encroach upon the space available for the emerging spinal nerve in the intervertebral foramen. This is the nature of nerve root involvement in cervical and lumbar spondylosis.

3 Cervical myelopathy (Chapter 10, see page 129) when **1**, or more commonly **2** above, causes spinal cord compression in the cervical region. This is more likely in patients with a constitutionally narrow spinal canal.

4 Cauda equina compression at several levels due to lumbar disc disease and spondylosis, often in association with a constitutionally narrow canal, may produce few or no neurological problems when the patient is at rest. The patient may develop sensory loss in the legs or weakness on exercise. This syndrome is not common, its mechanism is ill-understood, and it tends to be known as 'intermittent claudication of the cauda equina'.

Disc disease is confirmed by a combination of straight X-rays of the spine, CT scanning, and the use of water-soluble contrast material injected into the subarachnoid space (radiculography if only the cauda equina is to be visualized, myelography if the whole length of the spine is to be studied).

Most acute prolapsed discs settle spontaneously with rest and analgesics. Patients with marked signs of nerve root compression, with persistent symptoms despite adequate rest, or with recurrent symptoms, are probably best treated by surgical removal of the prolapsed material.

Cervical and lumbar spondylosis are difficult to treat satisfactorily, even when there are features of nerve root compression. Conservative treatment, analgesics, advice about bodyweight and exercise, use of collars and spinal supports are the more usual recommendations.

Spinal cord compression in the cervical region and severe cauda equina compression in the lumbar region may require surgical decompression by cervical or lumbar laminectomy.

Herpes zoster

Any sensory or dorsal root ganglion along the entire length of the neuraxis may be the site of active Herpes zoster infection. The painful vesicular eruption of shingles of dermatome distribution is well known. Pain may precede the eruption by a few days, secondary infection of the vesicles easily occurs, and pain may occasionally follow the rash on a long-term basis (post-herpetic neuralgia). The dermatome distribution of the shingles rash is one of the most dramatic living neuro-anatomical lessons to witness.

Occasionally, the Herpes zoster virus may enter the spinal

cord at the level of the infected dorsal root ganglion, causing lower motor neurone weakness at approximately the same level as the rash, or even a myelitis with long tract signs.

More about ophthalmic Herpes zoster infections appears in Chapter 3 (see page 41), and information about the nature of the infection, its significance, and treatment is given in Chapter 16 (see page 223).

Spinal tumours

Pain in the spine and nerve-root pain may indicate the presence of metastatic malignant disease in the spine. More occasionally, such pains may be due to a benign tumour such as a neurofibroma. The root pain may be either unilateral or bilateral. It is known as girdle pain when affecting the trunk, i.e. between T3 and L1. Segmental neurological signs in the form of lower motor neurone weakness, deep tendon reflex loss, and dermatome sensory abnormality may be evident, but the reason for early diagnosis and management is to prevent spinal cord compression, i.e. motor, sensory, and sphincter loss below the level of the lesion (Chapter 10, see pages 129 & 130). Treatment may involve surgery, radiotherapy, and chemotherapy in the case of metastatic disease, and will almost certainly involve successful surgery in the case of neurofibroma.

Brachial and lumbo-sacral plexus lesions

Lesions of these two nerve plexuses are not common, so they will be dealt with briefly. Of the two, brachial plexus lesions are the more common. In both instances, pain is a common symptom, together with sensory, motor and deep tendon reflex loss in the affected limb.

Spinal nerves from C5 to T1 contribute to the brachial plexus, which runs from the side of the lower cervical spine to the axilla, under the clavicle, and over the first rib and lung apex. Lesions of the brachial plexus are indicated in Fig. 13.6. A Horner's syndrome may be present if T1 is involved proximally (Chapter 12, see page 159 for details of the course of the sympathetic innervation of the eye).

Spinal nerves from L2 to S2 form the lumbo-sacral plexus, which runs downwards in the region of the ilio-psoas muscle, over the pelvic brim to the lateral wall of the pelvis. The only common pathology to affect this plexus is malignant disease, especially gynaecological cancer in females.

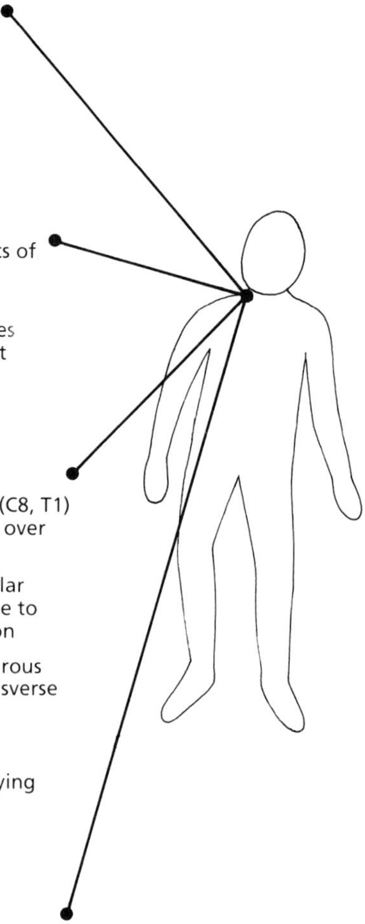

Trauma

Often very extensive damage

Usually a young man after a
  motor cycle injury

Disappointing recovery

Malignancy

Particularly apical lung cancer
  involving the lower elements of
  the plexus, known as the
  Pancoast tumour

As a consequence of metastases
  or of radiotherapy for breast
  cancer

Cervical rib

Lower elements of the plexus (C8, T1)
  are compressed as they pass over
  the rib to reach the axilla

There may be associated vascular
  insufficiency in the hand, due to
  subclavian artery compression

The 'rib' may be bone, or a fibrous
  band, running from the transverse
  process of C7 vertebra

More common in females

Symptoms aggravated by carrying
  anything heavy

Neuralgic amyotrophy

Uncommon patchy lesion of brachial
  plexus causing initial pain, followed
  by weakness, wasting, reflex and
  some sensory loss

Good prognosis

Fig. 13.6. Lesions of the brachial plexus.

Peripheral nerve lesions

Individual peripheral nerves in the limbs may be damaged
by any of five mechanisms:

1 *trauma:* in wounds created by sharp objects such as knives
or glass (e.g. median or ulnar nerve at the wrist), by
inaccurate localization of intramuscular injections (e.g.
sciatic nerve in the buttock), or by the trauma of bone
fractures (e.g. radial nerve in association with a midshaft
fracture of the humerus).

2 *acute compression:* in which pressure from a hard object is
exerted on a nerve. This may occur during sleep, anaesthesia, or coma in which there is no change in the position

of the body to relieve the compression (e.g. radial nerve compression against the posterior aspect of the humerus, common peroneal nerve against the lateral aspect of the neck of the fibula).

3 *iatrogenically:* following prolonged tourniquet application (e.g. radial nerve in the arm), or as a result of an ill-fitting plaster cast (e.g. common peroneal nerve in the leg).

4 *chronic compression:* so-called entrapment neuropathy, which occurs where nerves pass through confined spaces bounded by rigid anatomical structures, especially near to joints (e.g. ulnar nerve at the elbow or median nerve at the wrist).

5 as part of the clinical picture of *mononeuritis multiplex.* There are some conditions that can produce discrete focal lesions in individual nerves, so that the patient presents with more than one nerve palsy either simultaneously or consecutively (e.g. leprosy, diabetes, and polyarteritis nodosa).

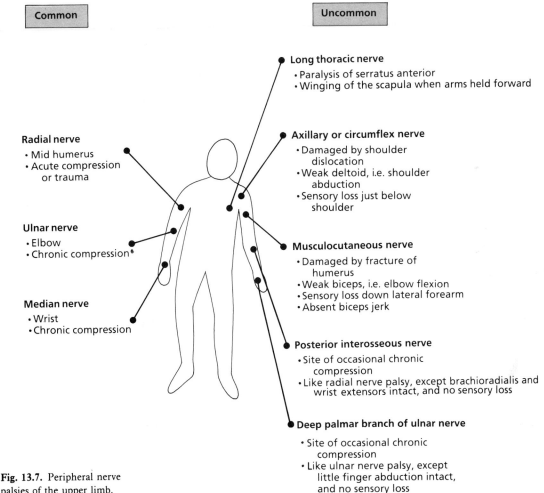

Common

Radial nerve
• Mid humerus
• Acute compression or trauma

Ulnar nerve
• Elbow
• Chronic compression *

Median nerve
• Wrist
• Chronic compression

Uncommon

Long thoracic nerve
• Paralysis of serratus anterior
• Winging of the scapula when arms held forward

Axillary or circumflex nerve
• Damaged by shoulder dislocation
• Weak deltoid, i.e. shoulder abduction
• Sensory loss just below shoulder

Musculocutaneous nerve
• Damaged by fracture of humerus
• Weak biceps, i.e. elbow flexion
• Sensory loss down lateral forearm
• Absent biceps jerk

Posterior interosseous nerve
• Site of occasional chronic compression
• Like radial nerve palsy, except brachioradialis and wrist extensors intact, and no sensory loss

Deep palmar branch of ulnar nerve
• Site of occasional chronic compression
• Like ulnar nerve palsy, except little finger abduction intact, and no sensory loss

Fig. 13.7. Peripheral nerve palsies of the upper limb.

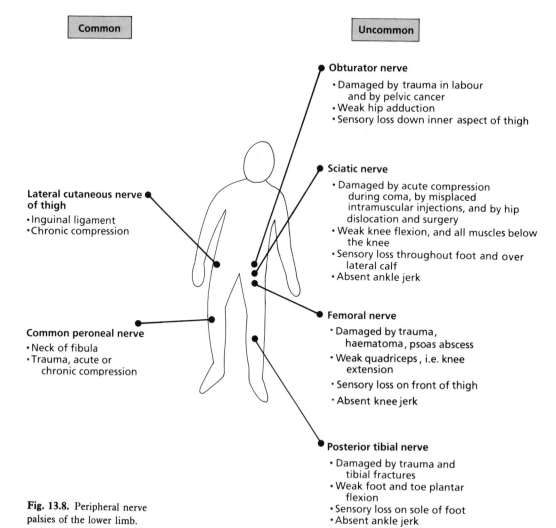

Obturator nerve
• Damaged by trauma in labour and by pelvic cancer
• Weak hip adduction
• Sensory loss down inner aspect of thigh

Sciatic nerve
• Damaged by acute compression during coma, by misplaced intramuscular injections, and by hip dislocation and surgery
• Weak knee flexion, and all muscles below the knee
• Sensory loss throughout foot and over lateral calf
• Absent ankle jerk

Lateral cutaneous nerve of thigh
• Inguinal ligament
• Chronic compression

Common peroneal nerve
• Neck of fibula
• Trauma, acute or chronic compression

Femoral nerve
• Damaged by trauma, haematoma, psoas abscess
• Weak quadriceps, i.e. knee extension
• Sensory loss on front of thigh
• Absent knee jerk

Posterior tibial nerve
• Damaged by trauma and tibial fractures
• Weak foot and toe plantar flexion
• Sensory loss on sole of foot
• Absent ankle jerk

Fig. 13.8. Peripheral nerve palsies of the lower limb.

Some peripheral nerve palsies are more common than others. Figures 13.7 and 13.8 show the common and uncommon nerve lesions in the upper and lower limbs, respectively. Brief notes about the uncommon nerve palsies are shown. The remainder of this chapter deals with the three common nerve palsies in the upper limbs and the two common ones in the legs.

Radial nerve palsy (Fig. 13.9)

The nerve is most usually damaged where it runs down the posterior aspect of the humerus in the spiral groove. This may occur as a result of acute compression, classically when a patient has gone to sleep with his arm hanging over the side of an armchair (Saturday night palsy!). It may occur in association with fractures of the midshaft of the humerus.

The predominant complaint is of difficulty in using the hand, because of wrist drop. The finger flexors and small hand muscles are greatly mechanically disadvantaged by the presence of wrist, thumb and finger extensor paralysis. There are usually no sensory complaints.

The prognosis is good after acute compression, and more variable after damage in association with a fractured humerus. The function of the hand can be helped by the use of a special 'lively' splint which holds the wrist, thumb and fingers in partial extension.

Fig. 13.9. Radial nerve palsy.

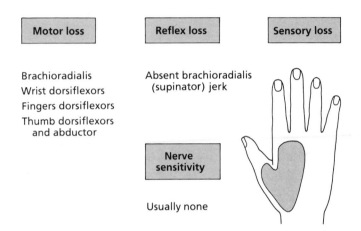

Motor loss	Reflex loss	Sensory loss

Brachioradialis
Wrist dorsiflexors
Fingers dorsiflexors
Thumb dorsiflexors
and abductor

Absent brachioradialis
(supinator) jerk

Nerve sensitivity

Usually none

Ulnar nerve palsy (Fig. 13.10)

The commonest aetiology is chronic compression, either in the region of the medial epicondyle, or a little more distally where the nerve enters the forearm between the two heads of flexor carpi ulnaris. Sometimes, the nerve is compressed acutely in this vicinity during anaesthesia or a period of enforced bedrest (during which the patient supports himself on the elbows whilst moving about in bed). The nerve may be damaged at the time of fracture involving the elbow, or subsequently if arthritic change or valgus deformity are the consequence of the fracture involving the elbow joint.

The patient complains of both motor and sensory symptoms, lack of grip in the hand, and painful paraesthesiae and numbness affecting the little finger and the ulnar border of the palm.

Persistent compression can be relieved by transposing the compressed nerve from behind to the front of the elbow joint. This produces good relief from the unpleasant sensory symptoms, and reasonable return of use of the hand even though there may be residual weakness and wasting of small hand muscles on examination.

185 *Peripheral nervous system*

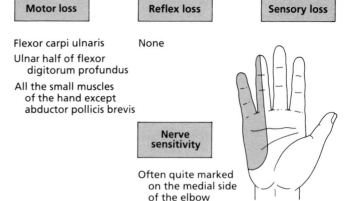

Motor loss	Reflex loss	Sensory loss
Flexor carpi ulnaris	None	
Ulnar half of flexor digitorum profundus		
All the small muscles of the hand except abductor pollicis brevis		

Nerve sensitivity

Often quite marked on the medial side of the elbow

Fig. 13.10. Ulnar nerve palsy.

Median nerve palsy (Fig. 13.11)

Carpal tunnel syndrome is the commonest clinical expression of median nerve palsy, and is probably the commonest nerve entrapment syndrome. The median nerve becomes chronically compressed within the carpal tunnel, which consists of the bony carpus posteriorly and the flexor retinaculum anteriorly. The carpal tunnel has a narrower cross-sectional area in women than men, and patients with carpal tunnel syndrome have a significantly narrower cross-sectional area in their carpal tunnels than a control population.

Carpal tunnel syndrome is five times more common in women than men. It is more common in patients who have arthritis involving the carpus, and is more frequent in pregnancy, diabetes, myxoedema, and acromegaly.

The patient complains of sensory symptoms. Painful paraesthesiae, swollen burning feelings, are felt in the affected hand and fingers, but often radiate above the wrist as high as the elbow. They frequently occur at night and interrupt sleep. They may occur after using the hands and arms. They are commonly relieved by shaking the arms. There are not usually any motor symptoms, except for possible impairment of manipulation of small objects between slightly numb thumb, index and middle fingers.

Symptomatic control may be established by wearing a wrist-immobilizing splint or by the use of hydrocortisone injection into the carpal tunnel. Permanent relief often requires surgical division of the flexor retinaculum, a highly effective and gratifying minor operation.

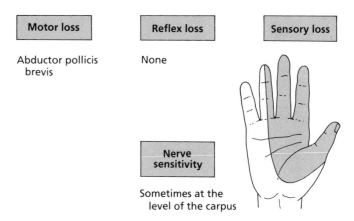

Motor loss	Reflex loss	Sensory loss
Abductor pollicis brevis	None	

Nerve sensitivity
Sometimes at the level of the carpus

Fig. 13.11. Median nerve palsy.

Meralgia paraesthetica

This irritating syndrome is the consequence of chronic entrapment of the lateral cutaneous nerve of thigh as it penetrates the inguinal ligament, or deep fascia, in the vicinity of the anterior superior iliac spine.

As the nerve is sensory, there are no motor symptoms. The patient complains of annoying paraesthesiae and partial numbness in a patch of skin on the antero-lateral aspect of the thigh (Fig. 13.12). The contact of clothes is slightly unpleasant in the affected area.

No treatment of meralgia paraesthetica may be necessary if the symptoms are mild. Alternatively, nerve decompression or section at the site of compression both give excellent relief.

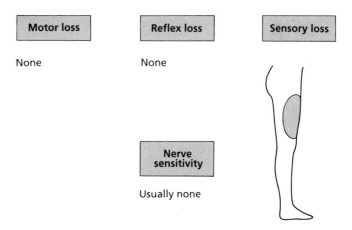

Motor loss	Reflex loss	Sensory loss
None	None	

Nerve sensitivity
Usually none

Fig. 13.12. Lateral cutaneous nerve of the thigh.

Common peroneal nerve palsy (Fig.13.13)

The common peroneal (lateral popliteal) nerve runs a very superficial course around the neck of the fibula. It divides into the peroneal nerve to supply the lateral calf muscles which evert the foot, and into the anterior tibial nerve which innervates the anterior calf muscles which dorsiflex the foot and toes. The nerve is liable to damage from trauma, with or without fracture of the fibula. It is highly susceptible to acute compression during anaethesia or coma, and from overtight or ill-fitting plaster casts applied for leg fractures.

The patient's predominant complaint is of foot drop, and the need to lift the leg up high when walking. He may complain of loss of normal feeling on the dorsal surface of the affected ankle and foot.

Treatment of common peroneal nerve palsy should be preventative wherever possible. A splint that keeps the ankle at a right angle may assist walking. The condition is not usually helped by any form of surgery.

Common peroneal nerve palsies due to acute compression have a good prognosis.

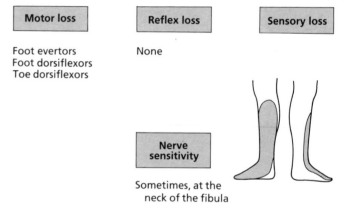

Motor loss	Reflex loss	Sensory loss
Foot evertors	None	
Foot dorsiflexors		
Toe dorsiflexors		

Nerve sensitivity

Sometimes, at the neck of the fibula

Fig. 13.13. Common peroneal nerve palsy.

Chapter 14

Motor neurone disease, peripheral neuropathy, myasthenia gravis and muscle disease

Introduction

This chapter is about the common disorders which affect the peripheral nervous system and muscle. They tend to produce a clinical picture of diffuse muscle weakness and wasting, and are sometimes a little difficult to distinguish from one another.

A diagrammatic summary of the four conditions under consideration appears in Fig. 14.1.

Fig. 14.1. The common peripheral neuromuscular disorders.

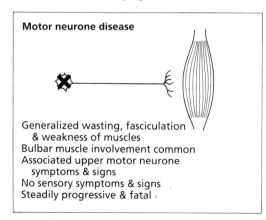

Motor neurone disease

Generalized wasting, fasciculation
  & weakness of muscles
Bulbar muscle involvement common
Associated upper motor neurone
  symptoms & signs
No sensory symptoms & signs
Steadily progressive & fatal

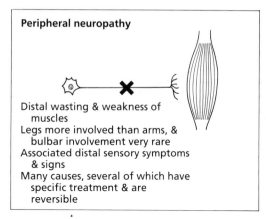

Peripheral neuropathy

Distal wasting & weakness of
  muscles
Legs more involved than arms, &
  bulbar involvement very rare
Associated distal sensory symptoms
  & signs
Many causes, several of which have
  specific treatment & are
  reversible

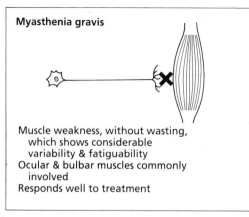

Myasthenia gravis

Muscle weakness, without wasting,
  which shows considerable
  variability & fatiguability
Ocular & bulbar muscles commonly
  involved
Responds well to treatment

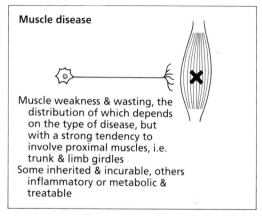

Muscle disease

Muscle weakness & wasting, the
  distribution of which depends
  on the type of disease, but
  with a strong tendency to
  involve proximal muscles, i.e.
  trunk & limb girdles
Some inherited & incurable, others
  inflammatory or metabolic &
  treatable

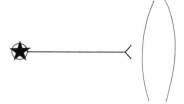

Motor neurone disease

This disease consists of a selective loss of lower motor neurones from the pons, medulla, and spinal cord, together with loss of upper motor neurones from the precentral gyri of the brain. The process is remarkably selective, leaving intelligence, special senses, cerebellar, sensory and autonomic functions intact. Progressive difficulty in doing things because of muscular weakness gradually overtakes the patient.

The cause of the neuronal loss in motor neurone disease (like the loss of neurones from other parts of the central nervous system, in diseases such as Alzheimer's and Parkinson's) is not understood.

There is variation in the clinical picture of motor neurone disease from one patient to another, which depends on:
• whether lower or upper motor neurones are predominantly involved;
• which muscles (bulbar, upper limb, trunk, or lower limb) are bearing the brunt of the illness;
• the rate of cell loss. Most usually, this is steadily progressive over a few years, but in a minority of cases it may be much more gradual with long survival.

Motor neurone disease tends to start either as a problem in the bulbar muscles, or as a problem in the limbs, and initially the involvement tends to be either lower motor neurone or upper motor neurone in nature. This has led to four clinical syndromes at the outset of the illness, which are described in Fig. 14.2.

As the illness progresses and the loss of motor neurones becomes more generalized, there is a tendency for both upper and lower motor neurone signs to become evident in bulbar, trunk and limb muscles. Sometimes, the illness may remain confined to the lower motor neurones, or to the upper motor neurones, but the co-existence of both, in the absence of sensory signs, is the hallmark of motor neurone disease. A limb with weak, wasted, fasciculating muscles, in which the deep tendon reflexes are very brisk, and in which there is no sensory loss, strongly suggests motor neurone disease.

It is the involvement of bulbar and respiratory muscles that is responsible for the inanition and chest infections which account for most of the deaths in patients with motor neurone disease.

There is no specific treatment for patients with motor neurone disease, yet patients can be helped by:
• humane explanation of the nature of the condition to the patient and his relatives;

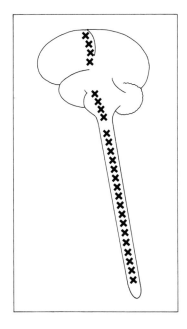

Fig. 14.2. The four clinical syndromes with which motor neurone disease may present.

Lower motor neurone	Upper motor neurone
Bulbar palsy	Pseudobulbar palsy
Bulbar muscle involvement	
Weakness, wasting and fasciculation of the lower facial muscles, and muscles moving the palate, pharynx, larynx, and tongue — most conspicuous in the tongue	Weakness, slowness and spasticity of the lower facial muscles, jaw, palate, pharynx, larynx and tongue muscles
	Exaggerated jaw jerk
	Emotional lability
Dysarthria, dysphagia, weight loss, and the risk of inhalation pneumonia are the clinical problems facing patients with either bulbar or pseudobulbar palsy	
Progressive muscular atrophy	Amyotrophic lateral sclerosis
Limb and trunk muscle involvement	
Weakness, wasting and fasciculation of any of the limb or trunk muscles	Weakness, spasticity, clonus and increased deep tendon reflexes
Often associated with frequent muscle cramps	Any limb, but more commonly in the legs
No sensory loss	Sphincter control not affected
Small muscles of the hand frequently involved	No sensory loss

- sympathy and encouragement;
- advice about diet in patients with dysphagia;
- speech therapy and communication aids in patients with dysarthria;
- provision of aids and alterations in the house (wheelchairs, ramps, lifts, showers, commodes, hoists, etc.) in time with their clinical deterioration;
- nursing help and respite care.

The lack of specific treatment should not lead to the feeling that there is nothing one can do for patients with motor neurone disease. They easily become socially isolated by their dysarthria, dysphagia, or limb paralysis. Regular medical attendance and organization of help is worthwhile and very much appreciated by the patient.

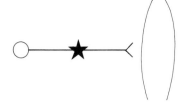

Peripheral neuropathy

In this section, we are focusing on the axon of the anterior horn cell and the distal axon of the dorsal root ganglion cell. These myelinated nerve fibres constitute the peripheral nerves (see Fig. 14.3). Each peripheral nerve, in reality, consists of very many myelinated nerve fibres.

In patients with peripheral neuropathy, there is malfunction in all the peripheral nerves of the body. The pathology may be distal axonal degeneration, but it is more usually a problem with the myelin along the whole course of the nerve. Segments of the nerve fibres become demyelinated (see Fig. 14.4). The normal saltatory passage of the nerve impulse along the nerve fibre becomes impaired. The impulse either fails to be conducted across the demyelinated section, or travels very slowly in a non-saltatory way along the axon in the demyelinated section of the nerve. This means that a large volley of impulses, which should travel synchronously along the component nerve fibres of a peripheral nerve, becomes:

• diminished as individual component impulses fail to be conducted;

• delayed and dispersed as individual impulses become slowed by the non-saltatory transmission (see Fig. 14.4).

Neurotransmission is most impaired in long nerves under such circumstances simply because the nerve impulse is confronted by a greater number of demyelinated segments

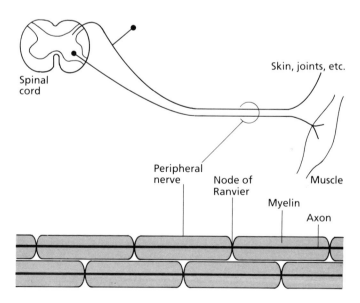

Fig. 14.3. Diagram to show the peripheral nerve components.

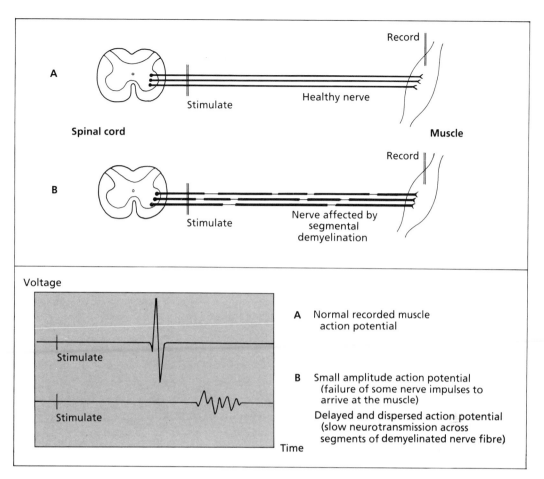

Record

A

Spinal cord

Stimulate

Healthy nerve

Muscle

Record

B

Stimulate

Nerve affected by
segmental
demyelination

Voltage

Stimulate

Stimulate

Time

A Normal recorded muscle
action potential

B Small amplitude action potential
(failure of some nerve impulses to
arrive at the muscle)

Delayed and dispersed action potential
(slow neurotransmission across
segments of demyelinated nerve fibre)

Fig. 14.4. Nerve conduction in healthy and segmentally demyelinated nerve fibres.

along the course of the nerve. This is the main reason why the symptoms of peripheral neuropathy are most evident distally in the limbs, why the legs and feet are more affected than the arms and hands, and why the distal deep tendon reflexes (which require synchronous neurotransmission from stretch receptors in the muscle to the spinal cord and back again to the muscle — the reflex arc) are frequently lost in patients with peripheral neuropathy.

Symptoms of peripheral neuropathy

The peripheral nerve pathology may predominantly affect sensory axons, motor axons or all axons. Thus, the patient's symptoms may be distal and sensory in the limbs (tingling, pins and needles, numbness, in a glove and stocking distribution). Alternatively patients may have muscle weakness and wasting in their hands for grip and fine finger movements, and in their lower legs and feet. The latter weakness may cause some degree of foot drop and lack of spring at the ankles for running and climbing stairs. The combination of distal sensory loss and weakness causes considerable clumsiness in the use of the fingers and hands for manipulation of buttons, coins, shoe-laces, knife and fork, keys, etc. In the legs and feet, the same combination of distal motor and sensory loss gives rise to unsteadiness of stance and gait, which is partially compensated by the use of the eyes. Eye closure (when washing, showering and dressing) and darkness may cause falls.

Common signs in peripheral neuropathy

The common physical signs in patients with peripheral neuropathy are:
- distal sensory loss affecting any modality, in the legs and hands;
- loss of distal deep tendon reflexes, particularly the ankle jerks;
- distal lower motor neurone signs in legs and hands.

Common causes of peripheral neuropathy

The common causes of peripheral neuropathy in the Western world are rather different from those worldwide. Deficiency of vitamin B_1 (dry beri-beri) and leprosy are the commonest causes of peripheral neuropathy in under-developed and equatorial countries. Figure 14.5 shows the commoner causes of peripheral neuropathy in the UK.

Alcoholic neuropathy

Alcoholic neuropathy is common and usually more sensory than motor. How much it is caused by the direct toxic effect of alcohol on the peripheral nerves, and how much it is due to co-existent vitamin B_1 deficiency, is not completely known.

Vitamin B_{12} deficiency

Vitamin B_{12} deficiency is not a common cause of neuropathy, but an important one to recognize because of its reversibility. Every effort should be made to reach the diagnosis before the irreversible changes of subacute combined degeneration of the spinal cord become established.

Diabetes mellitus

Diabetes mellitus is probably the commonest cause of peripheral neuropathy in the Western world. It occurs in

Deficiency	Vit. B_1 in alcoholics Vit. B_6 in patients taking isoniazid Vit. B_{12} in patients with pernicious anaemia and bowel disease
Toxic	Alcohol Drugs, e.g. isoniazid, vincristine, nitrofurantoin
Metabolic	Diabetes mellitus Chronic renal failure
Post-infective	Guillain-Barré syndrome
Paraneoplastic	Bronchial carcinoma and other malignancies
Collagen vascular disease	Rheumatoid arthritis Systemic lupus erythematosus Polyarteritis nodosa
Hereditary	Charcot-Marie-Tooth disease (also called peroneal muscular atrophy)
Idiopathic	Perhaps accounting for 50% of cases

Fig. 14.5. Common causes of peripheral neuropathy in the UK.

both juvenile-onset insulin-requiring diabetes and in maturity-onset diabetes. It may be the first clinical suggestion of the presence of diabetes. Evidence to support the prevention or improvement of neuropathy by excellent diabetic control is disappointingly marginal.

The commonest form of neuropathy in diabetes is a predominantly sensory one. The combination of neuropathy and atherosclerosis affecting the nerves and arteries in the lower limbs very strongly predisposes the feet of diabetic patients to trophic lesions, which are slow to heal.

There are a few unusual forms of neuropathy that may occur in patients with diabetes:
• a predominantly proximal neuropathy in the legs associated with pain, so-called diabetic amyotrophy;
• involvement of the autonomic nervous system giving rise to abnormal pupils, postural hypotension, impaired cardio-acceleration on changing from the supine to the standing position, impaired bladder, bowel and sexual function, and loss of normal sweating;
• a tendency for individual nerves to stop working quite abruptly, with subsequent gradual recovery. Common nerves to be involved are the 3rd, 6th and 7th cranial nerves and the common peroneal nerve in the leg. Involvement of several individual nerves in this way constitutes the clinical syndrome of mononeuritis multiplex.

195   *Peripheral neuromuscular disorders*

Guillain–Barré syndrome

Guillain–Barré syndrome is rather different to the other forms of peripheral neuropathy. This is because of its rapid evolution over several days, because it can produce a life-threatening degree of weakness, and because the underlying pathology clearly affects the nerve roots as well as the peripheral nerves.

The syndrome commonly occurs within two weeks of an infection, though sometimes no preceding infection can be identified. The patient notices limb weakness and sensory symptoms which worsen day by day for 1–2 weeks (occasionally the progression may continue for as long as 4 weeks). Often, the illness stops advancing after a few days and does not produce a disability that is too major. Not uncommonly, however, it progresses to cause very serious paralysis in the limbs, trunk and chest muscles, and in the muscles supplied by the cranial nerves. Patients with Guillain–Barré syndrome need to be hospitalized until it is certain that deterioration has come to an end, because chest and bulbar muscle weakness may make ventilation and nasogastric tube nutrition essential. Daily, or twice daily, estimations of the patient's vital capacity during the early phase of the disease can be a very valuable way of assessing the likelihood of the need for ventilatory support.

Patients with Guillain–Barré syndrome become very alarmed by the progressive loss of function at the start of their illness. They often need a good deal of psychological and physical support when the disability is severe and prolonged. The ultimate prognosis is usually very good however. Incomplete recovery and recurrence are both well described, but by far the most frequent outcome of this condition is complete recovery over a few weeks or months, and no further similar trouble thereafter.

The pathology is predominantly in the myelin rather than in the axons of the peripheral nerves and nerve roots, i.e. a demyelinating polyneuropathy and polyradiculopathy. The good overall prognosis is due to the fact that the majority of axons are intact, and recovery is due to the capability of Schwann cells to reconstitute the myelin sheaths after the initial demyelination. The involvement of the nerve roots gives rise to one of the diagnostic features of the condition, a raised CSF protein.

Peroneal muscular atrophy

Peroneal muscular atrophy is the commonest inherited peripheral neuropathy in the United Kingdom. The pattern of inheritance is usually of autosomal dominant type. The illness is usually evident in teenage life and very slowly worsens over many years. Motor involvement predominates, with lower motor neurone signs appearing in the feet and legs (especially in the antero-lateral muscle compartments of the calves), and in the small muscles of the hands. Pes cavus and clawing of the toes are very common consequences. Sometimes, the pathology involves the axons primarily, but more often there is demyelination and remyelination to be found in the peripheral nerves. Sometimes, the process of recurrent demyelination and remyelination is enough to thicken the nerves, so that they become more easily palpable than usual, e.g. the ulnar nerve at the elbow, and the common peroneal nerve at the neck of the fibula.

Myasthenia gravis

Myasthenia gravis is the rare clinical disease that results from impaired neuromuscular transmission at the synapse between the termination of the axon of the lower motor neurone and the muscle, at the motor end plate. Figure 14.6 is a diagram of a motor end plate. Neuromuscular transmission depends on normal synthesis and release of acetylcholine into the gap substance of the synapse, and its uptake by healthy receptors on the muscle membrane. In turn, this causes a rapidly travelling depolarization of the muscle membrane, associated with muscle contraction. The main pathological abnormality in myasthenia gravis at the neuromuscular junction is the presence of auto-antibody attached to receptor sites on the post-synaptic membrane, which reduces the number of acetycholine receptor sites available for neurotransmission across the synapse.

Myasthenia gravis is an auto-immune disease therefore, perhaps one of the best examples in clinical medicine since

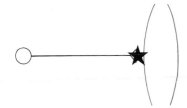

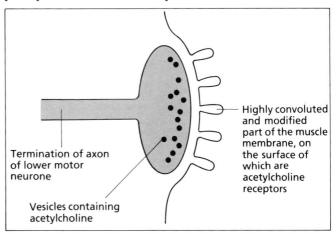

Termination of axon of lower motor neurone

Highly convoluted and modified part of the muscle membrane, on the surface of which are acetylcholine receptors

Vesicles containing acetylcholine

Fig. 14.6. Diagram to show a motor end plate in skeletal muscle.

the auto-antibody is so obviously involved in the disease process.

Myasthenia gravis is rather more common in women than men. In women, it tends to occur in young adult life, and in men it more commonly presents over the age of 50 years. Various subtypes of myasthenia gravis have been distinguished according to age and sex prevalence, HLA type associations, incidence of auto-antibodies, and other characteristics.

Muscle weakness with abnormal fatiguability and improvement after rest characterize myasthenia gravis. Symptoms tend to be worse at the end of the day, and after repetitive use of muscles for a particular task, e.g. chewing and swallowing may be much more difficult towards the end of a meal than they were at the start. The distribution of muscle involvement is not uniform, as indicated in Fig. 14.7.

	Muscles	Symptoms
Common	External ocular	Double vision and ptosis
	Bulbar	Difficulty in chewing, swallowing and talking
	Neck	Difficulty in lifting head up from the lying position
	Proximal limb	Difficulty in lifting arms above shoulder level, and in standing from low chairs and out of the bath
	Trunk	Breathing problems and difficulty in sitting from the lying position
Rare	Distal limb	Weak hand-grips, ankles and feet

Fig. 14.7. Frequency of muscle involvement and symptoms in myasthenia gravis.

Confirmation of the diagnosis

Once suspected, the diagnosis of myasthenia gravis may be confirmed by:
1 the Tensilon test. Edrophonium chloride (Tensilon) is a short-acting anticholinesterase, which prolongs the action of acetylcholine at the neuromuscular junction for a few minutes after intravenous injection. The patient is exercised in the part of the body which is showing myasthenic weakness, so that definite weakness is evident prior to injection. The rectifying effect of injection is usually striking to the patient and observers;

2 detection of circulating antibody to acetylcholine receptor site. This auto-antibody is not found in patients without myasthenia, and is found in approximately 90% of myasthenics;

3 electromyographic studies. Sometimes it is helpful to show that the amplitude of the compound muscle action potential, recorded by surface electrodes over a muscle, decreases on repetitive stimulation of the nerve to the muscle;

4 chest radiography and computerized tomography of the anterior mediastinum, to demonstrate an enlargement of the thymus gland. The association of myasthenia gravis with thymic enlargement is not yet fully understood. Of myasthenic patients, 10–15% have a thymoma, and 50–60% show 'thymitis'. Both sorts of pathology may enlarge the thymus, which can be clearly shown by suitable imaging procedures.

Management of myasthenia gravis

The management of myasthenia gravis includes:
1 the use of oral anticholinesterase drugs, pyridostigmine and prostigmine. These are prescribed at intervals during the day, and work quite effectively. Abdominal colic and diarrhoea, induced by the increased parasympathetic activity in the gut, can be controlled by simultaneous use of propantheline;

2 immuno-suppression by prednisone or azathioprine. In patients with disabling symptoms inadequately controlled by oral anticholinesterase therapy, suppression of the auto-antibody can radically improve muscle strength;

3 thymectomy. Remission or improvement can be expected in 60–80% of patients after thymectomy, and must be considered in all patients. It may make the use of immuno-suppressive drugs unnecessary, which is obviously desirable;

4 great care of the myasthenic patient with severe weakness who is already on treatment. The muscle strength of such patients may change abruptly, and strength in the bulbar and respiratory muscles may become inadequate for breathing. The correct place for such patients is in hospital, with anaesthetic and neurological expertise closely to hand. There may be uncertainty as to whether such a patient is under-treated with anticholinesterase (myasthenic crisis), or over-treated so that the excessive acetylcholine at the neuromuscular junction is spontaneously depolarizing the post-synaptic membrane, i.e. depolarization block (cholinergic crisis). Fasciculation may be present when such spontaneous depolarization is occurring. Tensilon may be used to decide whether the patient is under- or over-dosed, but *it is essential to perform the Tensilon test with an anaesthetist present in these circumstances*. If the weak state is due to cholinergic crisis, the additional intravenous dose of anticholinesterase may produce further critical paralysis of bulbar or respiratory muscles.

Muscle disease

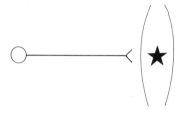

These are a group of rare diseases in which the primary pathology causing muscle weakness and wasting lies in the muscles themselves. They are classified in Fig. 14.8 and short notes about each condition are given in this section.

Inherited

1 Muscular dystrophies, in which the pathogenesis remains uncertain, though detection of the responsible gene is becoming possible, e.g.

Duchenne	X-linked recessive gene
Dystrophia myotonica	Autosomal dominant gene
Facio-scapulo-humeral	Autosomal dominant gene
Limb girdle	Not a single entity (variable inheritance)

2 Muscle diseases in which an inherited biochemical defect is present.

Specific enzyme deficiencies occur which *disrupt the pathways of carbohydrate or fat oxidation,* often with accumulation of substrate within the muscle cell. The enzyme deficiency may be within the muscle cell cytoplasm, interfering with the utilization of glycogen or glucose, or it may be within the mitochondria of muscle cells (and cells of other organs) blocking the metabolism of pyruvate, fatty acids or individual elements of Krebs cycle.

In other diseases of this sort, there is *uncoupling of the electrical excitation of muscle fibres and their contraction.* This is the case in McArdle's syndrome, and in malignant hyperpyrexia where sustained muscle contraction may occur in the absence of nerve stimulation.

Acquired

1 Immunologically mediated inflammatory disease, e.g.
   Polymyositis
   Dermatomyositis

2 Non-inflammatory myopathy, e.g.
   Corticosteroids
   Thyrotoxicosis

Fig. 14.8. Classification of muscle diseases.

Duchenne dystrophy

Duchenne dystrophy is the most serious inherited muscular dystrophy. The X-linked recessive inheritance gives rise to healthy female carriers and affected male children. The affected boys usually show evidence of muscular weakness before the age of 5 years, and die of profound muscle weakness (predisposing them to chest infections), or of associated cardiomyopathy, in late teenage life. In the early stages, the weakness of proximal muscles may show itself by a characteristic way in which these boys will 'climb up their own bodies with their hands' (Gower's sign) when rising from the floor to the standing position. They also show muscle wasting, together with pseudo-hypertrophy of the calf muscles (which is due to fat deposition in atrophied muscle tissue).

The affected boys have elevated levels of creatine phosphokinase and other muscle enzymes in the blood, and the clinically unaffected carrier state in female relatives is often associated with some elevation of the muscle enzymes in the blood. Recombinant DNA techniques now allow the identification of a genetic marker for Duchenne dystrophy on the X chromosome, a large region of DNA rather than a single gene.

This same region of the X chromosome is also implicated in the inheritance of a more benign variant of Duchenne dystrophy (later in onset and less rapidly progressive), known as Becker's muscle dystrophy.

The combination of family history, clinical examination, biochemical and chromosome studies allows the detection of the carrier state, and the pre-natal detection of the affected male fetus in the first trimester of pregnancy. Genetic counselling of such families has reached a high degree of accuracy.

Dystrophia myotonica

Dystrophia myotonica is characterized by 'dystrophy' of several organs and tissues of the body, and the dystrophic changes in muscle are associated with myotonic contraction.

The disease is transmitted by an autosomal dominant gene, so males and females are equally affected, usually in early adult life.

Some impairment of intellectual function, cataracts, premature loss of hair, cardiac arrhythmia and failure, gonadal atrophy and failure all feature in patients with dystrophia myotonica, but the most affected tissue is muscle. Muscle weakness and wasting are generalized, but facial, sternomastoid and hand muscles are very commonly involved.

The myotonia shows itself in two ways.

1 The patient has difficulty in rapid relaxation of tightly contracted muscle, contraction myotonia, and this is best seen by asking the patient to open the hand and fingers quickly after making a fist.

2 Percussion myotonia is the tendency for muscle tissue to contract when it is struck by a tendon hammer, and this is best seen by light percussion of the thenar eminence whilst the hand is held out flat. A sustained contraction of the thenar muscles lifts the thumb into a position of partial abduction and opposition.

From its appearance in early adult life, the illness runs a variable but slowly progressive course over several decades. The associated cardiomyopathy is responsible for some of the early mortality in dystrophia myotonica.

Some children of females with dystrophia myotonica may show the disease from the time of birth. Such babies may be very hypotonic, subject to respiratory problems (chest muscle involvement) and feeding problems (facial muscle involvement). Mental retardation is a feature of these children. Frequently, the birth of such a child is the first evidence of dystrophia myotonica in the family, since the mother's involvement is only mild.

A genetic marker for dystrophia myotonica has also been found. Clinical, biochemical and chromosome data allow accurate counselling and pre-natal testing in families with this condition.

Facio-scapulo-humeral dystrophy

Facio-scapulo-humeral dystrophy is generally a benign form of muscular dystrophy. It is of autosomal dominant inheritance, occurring in males and females. Its benign nature often allows the condition to be asymptomatic. Affected relatives with no symptoms may appear at the time of diagnosis of a patient in whom the condition is causing symptoms. Wasting and weakness of the facial, scapular, and humeral muscles may give rise to difficulties in whistling, and using the arms above shoulder level and for heavy lifting. The thinness of the biceps and triceps, or the abnormal position of the scapula (due to weakness of the muscles which hold the scapula close to the thoracic cage), may be the features that bring the patient to seek medical advice. Involvement of other trunk muscles, and the muscles of the pelvic girdle, may appear with time.

Limb girdle dystrophy

Limb girdle dystrophy is not a specific entity. There is an inherited muscle dystrophy with this distribution of weakness, but weakness of this sort may be caused by:

- muscle disease in which there is a specific biochemical defect;
- a rare and benign variant of motor neurone disease (chronic spinal muscular atrophy);
- polymyositis;
- myopathy in association with hormonal and metabolic disease.

Limb girdle weakness should not be regarded as dystrophy (and therefore untreatable), unless thorough investigation has shown this to be the case.

Conditions caused by inherited biochemical defects

Muscle diseases in which an inherited biochemical defect is present are rare, and require specialist expertise for confirmation. Of these conditions, malignant hyperpyrexia is perhaps the most dramatic. Members of families in which this condition is present do not have any ongoing muscle weakness or wasting. Symptoms do not occur until an affected family member has a general anaesthetic for surgery, particularly if halothane or suxamethonium chloride is used. During or immediately after surgery, muscle spasm, shock, and an alarming rise in body temperature occur, progressing to death in about 50% of cases.

The pathology of this condition involves a defect in calcium metabolism allowing such anaesthetic agents to incur a massive rise in calcium ions within the muscle cells. This is associated with sustained muscle contraction and muscle necrosis. The rise in body temperature is secondary to the generalized muscle contraction.

Polymyositis and dermatomyositis

In polymyositis and dermatomyositis, the condition of the muscles is identical. There is a mononuclear inflammatory cell infiltration and muscle fibre necrosis. In dermatomyositis, there is the additional involvement of skin, particularly in the face and hands. An erythematous rash over the nose and around the eyes, and over the knuckles of the hands, is most typical. Though all muscles may be involved, proximal limb, trunk, and neck muscles are most frequently made weak by polymyositis with occasional involvement of swallowing.

The condition most usually develops subacutely or chronically and is unassociated with muscle tenderness. Problems when trying to use the arms above shoulder level, and difficulty when standing up out of low chairs and the bath, are the most frequent complaints.

Polymyositis is an auto-immune disease involving skeletal and not cardiac muscle, and sometimes occurs in association with malignant disease (especially dermatomyositis in males over 45 years of age).

Both dermatomyositis and polymyositis respond to immuno-suppressive therapy. High-dose steroids, with or without azathioprine, gradually reduced to reasonable long-term maintenance levels, constitute the treatment of choice. Effective control of the disease can be established in the majority of cases.

Acquired non-inflammatory myopathy

Acquired non-inflammatory myopathy can occur in many circumstances (alcoholism, drug-induced states, disturbances of vitamin D and calcium metabolism, Addison's disease, etc.), but the two common conditions to be associated with myopathy are *hyperthyroidism* and *high-dose steroid treatment*.

Many patients with hyperthyroidism show weakness of shoulder girdle muscles. This is usually asymptomatic. Occasionally, more serious weakness of proximal limb muscles and trunk muscles may occur. The myopathy completely recovers with treatment of the primary condition.

Patients on high-dose steroids, especially the fluorinated triamcinolone, betamethasone, and dexamethasone, may develop significant trunk and proximal limb muscle weakness and wasting. The myopathy is reversible on withdrawal of the steroids, on reduction in dose, or on change to a non-fluorinated steroid.

The investigation of patients with generalized muscle weakness and wasting

The last section of this chapter discusses the common investigations that are carried out in patients with generalized muscle weakness and wasting. Of the four conditions discussed in this chapter, myasthenia gravis does not produce muscle wasting, and is usually distinguishable by virtue of the ocular and bulbar muscle involvement, the abnormal degree of fatiguability, and the response to anticholinesterase. The other three conditions may be

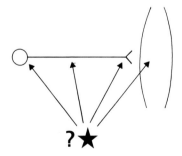

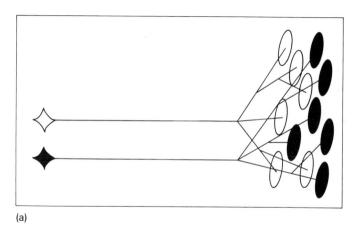

(a)

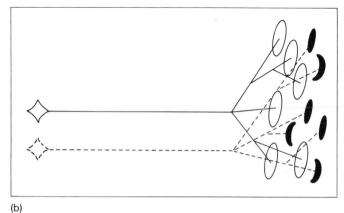

Fig. 14.9. The changes in denervation. (a) Two normal motor units. Each lower motor neurone supplies several muscle fibres. (b) Damage to one lower motor neurone, either in the cell body (as in motor neurone disease), or in the axon (as in peripheral neuropathy), results in denervated muscle fibres within the motor unit. (c) The surviving lower motor neurone produces terminal axonal sprouts which innervate some of the muscle fibres of the damaged motor unit. Therefore, in muscles affected by a denervating disease, there is *a reduced number of abnormally large motor units.*

(b)

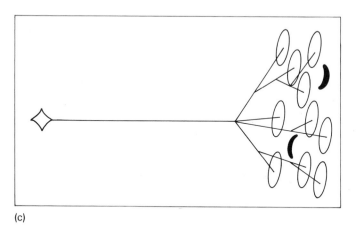

(c)

quite distinct on clinical grounds too, but investigation is frequently very helpful in confirmation of diagnosis.

It is important that the consequences of denervation and muscle disease on the motor unit are understood, and these are shown in Figs 14.9 and 14.10. Both electromyography (the recording of muscle at rest and during contraction) and muscle biopsy are able to detect the classical changes of

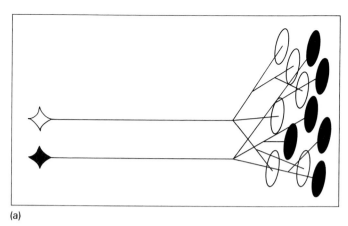

(a)

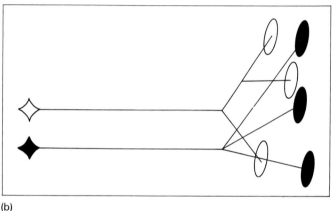

(b)

Fig. 14.10. The changes of muscle disease. (a) Two normal motor units. Each lower motor neurone supplies several muscle fibres. (b) In muscle disease (dystrophy, polymyositis, or acquired myopathy), there is loss or damage directly affecting muscle fibres. The number of functional muscle fibres decreases. Therefore, in muscle disease, there is *a normal number of abnormally small motor units.*

chronic partial denervation (a reduced number of abnormally large motor units), and of primary muscle disease (a normal number of abnormally small motor units).

Figure 14.11 shows the triad of investigations that is carried out on patients of this sort.

Of the conditions considered in this chapter, significant elevation of muscle enzymes occurs only in muscle disease, in which the primary insult is to the muscle fibres, resulting in leakage of their contents into the blood. (Other causes of muscle necrosis, e.g. crush injury, status epilepticus, may also produce high levels of muscle enzymes in the blood.)

Electromyography is good in differentiating denervation from muscle disease, as already mentioned. In patients in whom denervation is found, nerve conduction studies will differentiate nerve cell body disease, e.g. motor neurone disease, in which conduction is quite normal in the surviving axons, from neuropathy, in which the pathology is in the myelinated axons with consequent slowing of conduction.

Muscle biopsy differentiates denervation from muscle disease well, and gives further specific commentary on the nature of the muscle disease. There are characteristic features of dystrophy, polymyositis and acquired myopathy.

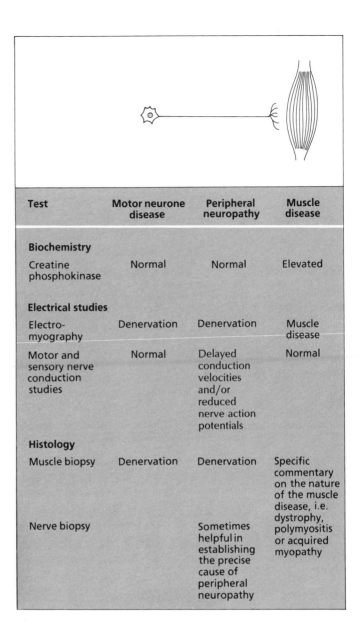

Test	Motor neurone disease	Peripheral neuropathy	Muscle disease
Biochemistry			
Creatine phosphokinase	Normal	Normal	Elevated
Electrical studies			
Electro-myography	Denervation	Denervation	Muscle disease
Motor and sensory nerve conduction studies	Normal	Delayed conduction velocities and/or reduced nerve action potentials	Normal
Histology			
Muscle biopsy	Denervation	Denervation	Specific commentary on the nature of the muscle disease, i.e. dystrophy, polymyositis or acquired myopathy
Nerve biopsy		Sometimes helpful in establishing the precise cause of peripheral neuropathy	

Fig. 14.11. The triad of investigations in patients with generalized muscle weakness and wasting, and the results found in the three common causes.

Light and electron microscopy, histochemistry and im-muno-fluorescent techniques are all applied to the biopsied muscle tissue to provide a high degree of diagnostic accuracy.

Chapter 15　Disorders of talking and walking

Speech disorders

Introduction

A common reaction to meeting someone who is unable to speak properly is to think that the person is intellectually subnormal, mad, or drunk. Patients with speech disorders worry that their abnormal speech might be interpreted in one of these ways. Dysphasic patients, in whom there is profound loss of language comprehension, are not infrequently referred to psychiatric units before the real nature of their problem is recognized. Patients with cerebellar dysarthria are very aware that their speech sounds like the speech of alcoholic intoxication.

Understanding speech disorders will help to guard against such hasty judgements. This chapter will not cover impaired speech development in childhood (resulting from deafness, mental retardation, adverse psychological and social factors), nor will it comment on the problem of stuttering. The chapter is mainly concerned with the three broad ways in which speech and language may become impaired in adult life, having been previously normal.

Dysphasia

Patients with dysphasia have a language problem. This is not dissimilar to being in a foreign country and finding oneself unable to understand what is being said on the one hand, and being unable to express oneself to other people on the other.

Figure 15.1 sets out the two main types of dysphasia (as seen in the majority of people, in whom speech is represented in the left cerebral hemisphere). Not infrequently, a patient has a lesion in the left cerebral hemisphere which is large enough to produce a global or mixed dysphasia. Broca's and Wernicke's areas are both involved, verbal expression and comprehension are both impaired.

Involvement of nearby areas of the brain by the lesion

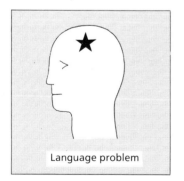

Language problem

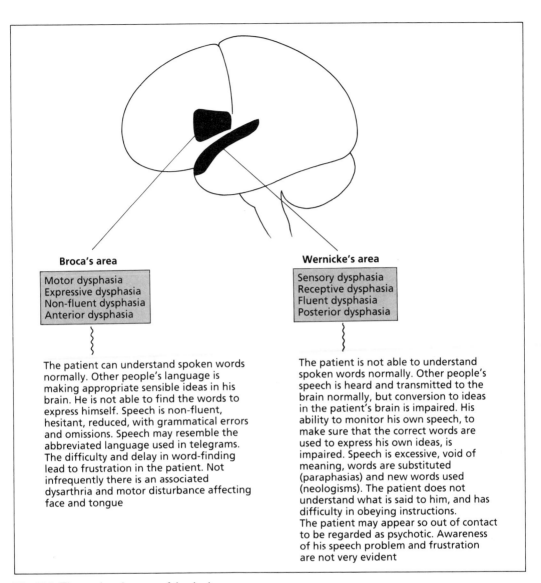

Broca's area

Motor dysphasia
Expressive dysphasia
Non-fluent dysphasia
Anterior dysphasia

The patient can understand spoken words normally. Other people's language is making appropriate sensible ideas in his brain. He is not able to find the words to express himself. Speech is non-fluent, hesitant, reduced, with grammatical errors and omissions. Speech may resemble the abbreviated language used in telegrams. The difficulty and delay in word-finding lead to frustration in the patient. Not infrequently there is an associated dysarthria and motor disturbance affecting face and tongue

Wernicke's area

Sensory dysphasia
Receptive dysphasia
Fluent dysphasia
Posterior dysphasia

The patient is not able to understand spoken words normally. Other people's speech is heard and transmitted to the brain normally, but conversion to ideas in the patient's brain is impaired. His ability to monitor his own speech, to make sure that the correct words are used to express his own ideas, is impaired. Speech is excessive, void of meaning, words are substituted (paraphasias) and new words used (neologisms). The patient does not understand what is said to him, and has difficulty in obeying instructions.
The patient may appear so out of contact to be regarded as psychotic. Awareness of his speech problem and frustration are not very evident

Fig. 15.1. The two broad groups of dysphasia.

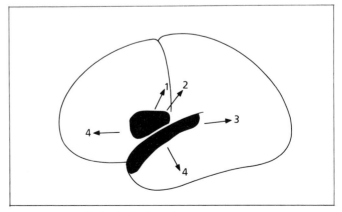

1 Weakness of the right face, hand and arm

2 Sensory impairment in the right face, hand and arm

3 Difficulties with:
   written words . . . dyslexia and dysgraphia
   numbers . . . dyscalculia
   visual field . . . right homonymous hemianopia

4 Impairment of memory, alteration of behaviour

Fig. 15.2. The common associated neurological abnormalities in dysphasic patients.

causing the dysphasia may result in other clinical features. These are shown in Fig. 15.2. Stroke, ischaemic or haemorrhagic, and cerebral tumour are the common sorts of focal pathology to behave in this way.

Dysarthria

The speech disturbance in patients with dysarthria is a purely mechanical one caused by defective movement of the lips, tongue, palate, pharynx, and larynx. Clear pronunciation of words is impaired due to the presence of a neuromuscular lesion.

Speaking is a complex motor function. Like complex movement of other parts of the body, normal speech requires the integrity of basic components of the nervous system, mentioned in Chapter 5, and illustrated again in Fig. 15.3. There are characteristic features of the speech when there is a lesion in each element of the nervous system identified in Fig. 15.3. These are the different types of dysarthria.

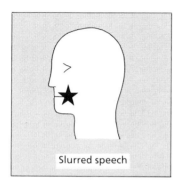

Slurred speech

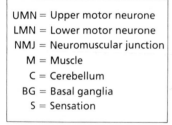

UMN = Upper motor neurone
LMN = Lower motor neurone
NMJ = Neuromuscular junction
M = Muscle
C = Cerebellum
BG = Basal ganglia
S = Sensation

Fig. 15.3. Basic components of the nervous system required for normal movement.

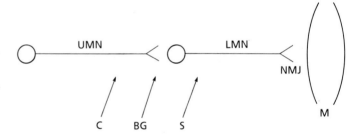

Upper motor neurone lesions

The upper motor neurones involved in speech have their cell bodies at the lower end of the precentral (motor) gyrus in each cerebral hemisphere. From the motor cortex, the axons of these cells descend via the internal capsule to the contralateral cranial nerve nuclei 5, 7, 9, 10, and 12, as shown in Fig. 15.4.

A unilateral lesion does not usually produce a major problem of speech pronunciation. There is some slurring of speech due to facial weakness in the presence of a hemiparesis.

Bilateral upper motor neurone lesions, on the other hand, nearly always produce a significant speech disturbance. Weakness of the muscles supplied by cranial nerves 5–12 is known as bulbar palsy if the lesion is lower motor neurone in type (see the next section in this chapter). It is known as

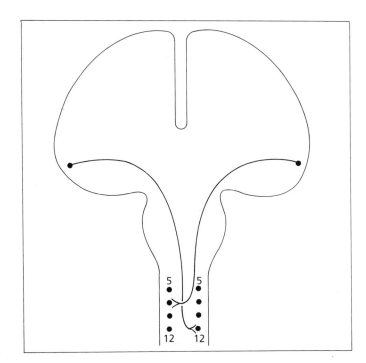

Fig. 15.4. The upper and lower motor neurones involved in speech.

pseudobulbar palsy if the weakness is upper motor neurone in type. Patients who have bilateral upper motor neurone weakness of their lips, jaw, tongue, palate, pharynx, and larynx, i.e. patients with pseudobulbar palsy, have a characteristic speech disturbance, known as a spastic dysarthria. The speech is slow, indistinct, laboured, and stiff. Muscle wasting is not present, the jaw jerk is increased, and there may be associated emotional lability. The patient is likely to be suffering from bilateral cerebral hemisphere cerebrovascular disease, motor neurone disease, or serious multiple sclerosis.

Lower motor neurone lesions, and lesions in the neuromuscular junction and muscles

The lower motor neurones involved in speech have their cell bodies in the pons and medulla (Fig. 15.4), and their axons travel out to the muscles of the jaw, lips, tongue, palate, pharynx, and larynx in cranial nerves 5–12.

A single unilateral cranial nerve lesion does not usually produce a disturbance of speech, except in the case of 7. A severe unilateral facial palsy does cause some slurring of speech.

Multiple unilateral cranial nerve lesions are very rare (e.g. in posterior inferior cerebellar artery occlusion, and other rare conditions), but do interfere with speech clarity.

Bilateral weakness of the bulbar muscles, whether pro-

211 *Disorders of talking and walking*

duced by pathology in the lower motor neurones, neuro-muscular junction, or muscles, is known as bulbar palsy. One of the predominant features of bulbar palsy is the disturbance of speech. The other main features are difficulty in swallowing and incompetence of the larynx leading to aspiration pneumonia. The speech is quiet, indistinct, with a nasal quality if the palate is weak, poor gutturals if the pharynx is weak, and poor labials if the lips are weak. (Such a dysarthria may be rehearsed if one tries to talk without moving lips, palate, throat, and tongue.)

Motor neurone disease, Guillain–Barré syndrome, and myasthenia gravis all cause bulbar palsy due to lesions in the cranial nerve nuclei, cranial nerve axons, and neuromuscular junctional regions of the bulbar muscles, respectively (Chapter 12, page 171 and Fig. 12.14).

Cerebellar lesions

As already mentioned, the dysarthria of patients with cerebellar disease often embarrasses them because their speech sounds as if they are drunk. There is poor coordination of muscular action, of agonists, antagonists and synergists. There is ataxia of the speaking musculature, very similar to the limb ataxia seen in patients with cerebellar lesions. Speech is irregular, both in volume and timing. It is referred to as a scanning or staccato dysarthria.

Drugs that affect cerebellar function (alcohol, anticonvulsants), multiple sclerosis, cerebrovascular disease, and posterior fossa tumours are some of the more common causes of cerebellar malfunction.

Basal ganglion lesions

The bradykinesia of Parkinson's disease causes the characteristic dysarthria of this condition. The speed and amplitude of movements are reduced. Speech is quiet, indistinct, and lacks up and down modulation. A monotonous voice from a fixed face, both voice and face lacking lively expression, is the typical state of affairs in Parkinson's disease.

Patients with chorea may have sudden interference of their speech if a sudden involuntary movement occurs in their respiratory, laryngeal, mouth, or facial muscles.

Sensory lesions

Speech disorders secondary to sensory loss do not occur very often. (Talking is slightly difficult after a quarter of the mouth has been made anaesthetic at the dentist's surgery!)

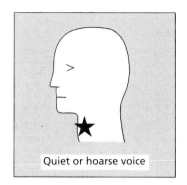

Quiet or hoarse voice

Dysphonia

Voice production requires the passage of air past the vocal cords in the larynx. The voice may become weak or hoarse if the chest muscles are weak, if the movements of the vocal cords are weak, or if the vocal cords are diseased.

Local disease of the vocal cords is the commonest cause of dysphonia, e.g. laryngitis, nodules or carcinoma affecting the vocal cords.

Weakness of one vocal cord occurs in a recurrent laryngeal nerve palsy and causes hoarseness.

More generalized weakness of chest muscles and larynx occurs in motor neurone disease, Guillain–Barré neuropathy, myasthenia gravis, and primary muscle disease. In such cases, dysphonia may co-exist with dysarthria due to associated bulbar muscle weakness.

Gait disorders

Introduction

Not all abnormalities of gait are due to neurological disease. Joint disease, especially when affecting the hip and knee, and painful conditions of the foot, commonly alter the way in which a patient walks. From the neurological point of view, important diagnostic information may be evident as the patient walks into the consulting room. It is unsatisfactory if patients with neurological disorders have to be interviewed and examined in a confined space, because this does not allow proper attention to the gait.

Those interested in communication between individuals by non-verbal signals would emphasize that one can obtain some idea of a patient's feelings about his illness by watching him walk. For instance, determination, embarrassment, frustration, lack of confidence, self-pity, etc. may be very evident in the gait of a paraparetic or hemiparetic patient.

With experience, it is sometimes possible to know what is the matter with the patient, and to have some idea of how he is coping with it, simply by watching him walk into the consulting room and sit down.

Not every neurological gait is discussed in this chapter. The common ones are described, using the same diagrammatic model for movement as mentioned in Chapter 5, and in the first half of this chapter, when considering dysarthria (Fig. 15.3).

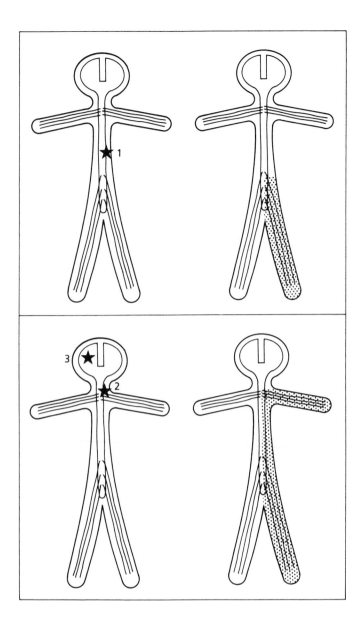

Fig. 15.5. Unilateral upper motor neurone lesions affecting gait: **1** in the spinal cord below the cervical region; **2** in the upper cervical region of the spinal cord; **3** in the cerebral hemisphere.

Upper motor neurone lesions

Upper motor neurone lesions are illustrated in Figs 15.5 and 15.6.

A unilateral lesion in the spinal cord below the neck (Fig. 15.5 1) produces upper motor neurone weakness of one leg. As the patient walks, both arms and the other leg are normal. The affected leg is stiff due to increased tone, and tends to drag and catch the toes as the foot is moved forward. This is because of the weakness of hip flexion, knee flexion, and foot dorsiflexion which are predominant in upper motor neurone weakness of the leg.

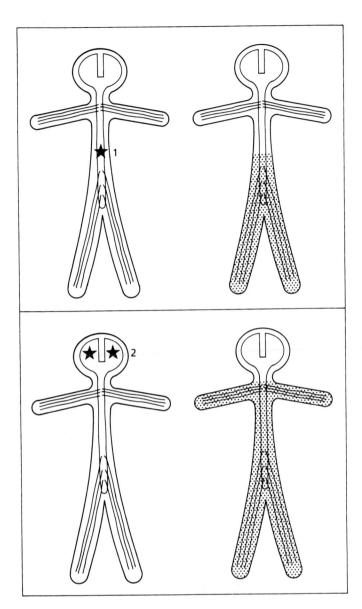

Fig. 15.6. Bilateral upper motor neurone lesions affecting gait: **1** in the spinal cord; **2** in the cerebral hemispheres.

A unilateral high cervical cord lesion (Fig. 15.5 **2**), or a contralateral cerebral hemisphere lesion (Fig. 15.5 **3**), causes the same abnormality of the leg when walking, but the arm does not move normally during walking. There is a tendency to adduction of the arm against the body at the shoulder, and the forearm is held across the body due to flexion at the elbow and pronation of the forearm. This is the classical posture of the arm during walking in the presence of an upper motor neurone lesion.

Bilateral upper motor neurone weakness of the legs is most commonly due to a lesion in the spinal cord, as shown in Fig. 15.6 **1**. Both legs are stiff. They move forward slowly

215   *Disorders of talking and walking*

and with obvious effort (due to the weakness of hip flexion) with bilateral scuffing of the toes (due to the ankle dorsiflexion weakness). There may be some tendency to adduction of the legs at the hips.

When there is damage to the upper motor neurones in both cerebral hemispheres early in life (Fig. 15.6 2), the child grows up with a spastic diplegia. All four limbs are stiff, both arms are adducted at the shoulders, and flexed and pronated at the elbow and wrist. The increase in tone in the legs not infrequently causes some permanent flexion and adduction at the hips as the patient walks, with some knee flexion and fixed foot plantar flexion. The adduction at the hip and tendency to walk on the toes are very characteristic features of the spastic person's gait. The disability is frequently not symmetrical.

Lower motor neurone lesions

Patients with nerve root problems (Fig. 15.7 1) in the lumbosacral region may walk abnormally. Since such lesions are usually due to prolapsed intervertebral discs, they are most commonly unilateral and often painful. The pain of the lumbago and sciatica may modify the gait. The body leans away from the side of the disc problem, and weight-bearing on the painful leg produces a limp. In addition, there may be gait abnormality because of muscular weakness due to motor root compression:
• weakness of foot plantar-flexion occurs with Sl root lesions. This produces lack of spring at the ankle when walking, and inability to stand and walk on tiptoe;
• L4/5 weakness produces weakness of foot and toe dorsi-flexion, so that the patient walks with a foot drop. To clear the ground as the foot moves forward, there has to be unnatural elevation of the knee, during which the forefoot tends to hang. The patient is unable to walk on his heels, the forefoot on the affected side refusing to come off the ground;
• L2/3/4 root lesions, which are less common, produce weakness of the quadriceps. This makes the knee very susceptible to giving way, especially when walking down-stairs (which normally requires the bodyweight to be supported on a partially flexed knee, as each downward step is taken).

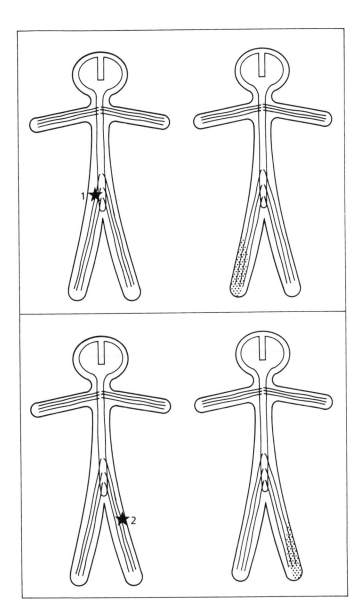

Fig. 15.7. Unilateral lower motor neurone lesions affecting gait: **1** in a nerve root, e.g. L5; **2** in a peripheral nerve, e.g. common peroneal nerve.

The most common single peripheral nerve lesion to produce a gait abnormality is a common peroneal (lateral popliteal) nerve palsy (Fig. 15.7 **2**). This produces a foot drop, difficult to differentiate from an L4/5 nerve root lesion. The same unnatural elevation of the knee occurs as the affected leg moves forward, the same hanging of the forefoot, and a tendency for the toes to hit the ground before the heel as the weight is transferred onto the affected foot. This sometimes introduces an audible 'double-strike' abnormality to the gait.

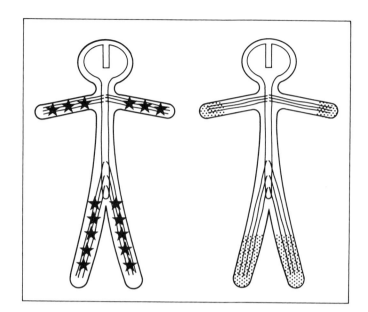

Fig. 15.8. Bilateral lower motor neurone lesions affecting gait: peripheral neuropathy.

Peripheral neuropathy (Fig. 15.8) is the commonest cause of bilateral lower motor neurone weakness in the legs to cause gait disturbance. The weakness is most marked distally so that the patient walks with bilateral foot drop and bilateral lack of spring at the ankles, due to weakness of all muscles below the knees. He is unable to walk on tiptoe or on his heels. There may be associated sensory loss in the feet, so that the patient has to watch the floor and his feet carefully as he walks. This sensory aspect is described later in the chapter.

Muscle disease

Proximal muscle weakness typifies most primary muscle disease. When marked, the weakness of the trunk and pelvic girdle muscles produces a stereotyped gait disturbance. The patient has difficulty in rising from a chair into the standing

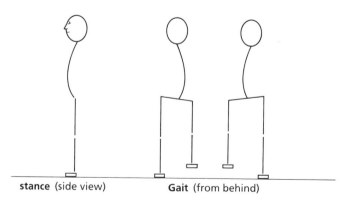

stance (side view)   **Gait** (from behind)

Fig. 15.9. Proximal muscle weakness affecting stance and gait.

position. He needs to use his arms to help him do this. In the standing position, the trunk muscle weakness often allows an abnormal amount of extension of the lumbar spine, so that the abdomen protrudes forwards. When walking, the abdominal and pelvic muscle weakness allows downward tilting of the pelvis when the leg is off the ground, as shown in Fig. 15.9. This is known as Trendelenburg weakness.

Cerebellar disorders

Unsteadiness of gait is a common manifestation of a lesion in the cerebellum, or of a lesion in the brainstem affecting cerebellar input or outflow.

With a lateralized cerebellar or brainstem lesion, there is deviation and impaired balance towards the side of the lesion.

With a midline cerebellar lesion, there is gait unsteadiness without lateralization, sometimes unassociated with many other abnormal cerebellar signs.

Basal ganglion disorders

Patients with Parkinson's disease adopt a posture of slight universal flexion in the standing position. They walk with small, shuffling steps and with reduced swinging of the arms. There is frequently difficulty in starting and stopping, and a tendency to shuffle badly when turning and in confined spaces. Walking up and down stairs is sometimes remarkably good, even when walking on the flat is profoundly affected. Balance is poor because of bradykinesia, body rigidity, and impaired postural reflexes. Tremor, or dopamine-induced involuntary movements, may be quite conspicuous as the patient walks.

The sudden involuntary movements which occur in patients with Huntington's chorea may be a marked feature of the gait, and Sydenham's chorea was also known as St Vitus' dance. Sometimes, the movements are sudden enough to cause falls.

Sensory deficits

The three main places where lesions may occur in the nervous system to cause sensory loss that affects gait are shown in Figs 15.10 and 15.11.

Lesions in the parietal lobe may cause sensory inattention and sensory loss in the contralateral limbs (Fig. 15.10). Patients tend to ignore the affected side of the body. They forget to move it automatically when getting to their feet,

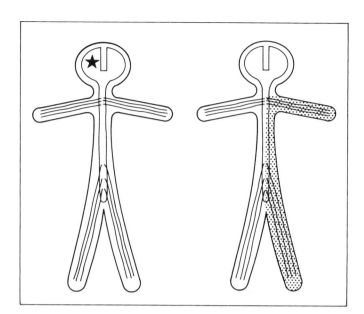

Fig. 15.10. Sensory deficits affecting gait: cerebral hemisphere lesion.

and may bump into furniture or door-posts on the affected side (especially if there is associated contralateral visual field inattention or loss).

Loss of proprioceptive sense in the legs and feet may occur either as a result of spinal cord disease (Fig. 15.11 **1**), or peripheral neuropathy (Fig. 15.11 **2**). The loss of sense of position gives rise to clumsiness of leg movement when walking, unsteadiness, the need to watch the feet and floor carefully, and marked unsteadiness and falling when vision cannot compensate, e.g. in the dark, in the shower, when washing the face, when putting clothes over the head. Romberg's sign (stance steady with eyes open, but unsteady with eyes closed) is positive in such patients.

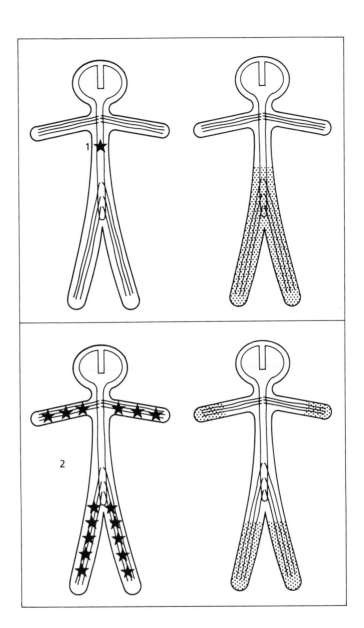

Fig. 15.11. Sensory deficits affecting gait: 1 spinal cord lesion; 2 peripheral neuropathy.

Chapter 16

Infections of the nervous system

Introduction

The human nervous system can be infected by:
- parasites (hydatid cysts and cysticercosis);
- protozoa (*toxoplasma*);
- *Rickettsii* (Rocky Mountain spotted fever);
- mycoplasma (*Mycoplasma pneumoniae*);
- spirochaetes (syphilis, leptospirosis, etc.);
- fungi (*Cryptococcus, Candida* , etc.);
- chronic mycobacteria (tuberculosis and leprosy);
- pyogenic bacteria (*Haemophilus influenzae*, meningo-coccus, etc.);
- chronic viruses (AIDS, SSPE, etc.);
- acute viruses (Herpes simplex and Herpes zoster, poliovirus, etc.);
- probable infective agents smaller than viruses, yet to be identified (kuru and Jakob–Creutzfeldt disease).

In this chapter, we will try to simplify our understanding of such a large area of neurological disease, identifying the features that many of these infections have in common. We will pay most attention to those that are already common in the UK, or which are becoming more common in the late twentieth century.

Common localized infections

Viral infections

Some viruses have a predilection for particular elements of the nervous system. The common ones are illustrated in Fig. 16.1 next to the relevant description on p.223.

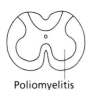

Poliomyelitis

Acute poliomyelitis

Acute poliomyelitis is uncommon in the UK nowadays, but only as a result of the highly developed immunization programme. When polio does occur, it is in members of the community who have escaped immunization (e.g. gypsies), or in people who have been abroad to a part of the world where the disease is much more prevalent, who have not had any recent 'booster' to their polio immunization status.

After a gastro-enterological infection, the virus takes up residence in lower motor neurones (in the spinal cord and brainstem). Paralysis ensues, which is often patchy and asymmetrical in the body. Where the infection has been very severe in the neuraxis, lower motor neurones do not recover and the paralysis is permanent. Some of the damage to lower motor neurones is less complete, and frequently there is recovery of some muscle function after a few weeks.

Rehabilitation and orthopaedic treatment may be necessary to make the most of residual function after poliomyelitis.

Herpes zoster,
Herpes simplex, type 2

Herpes zoster infections

Herpes zoster infections, or *shingles*, have been described in Chapters 3 (page 41), 12 (page 162) and 13 (page 180). The virus probably enters the dorsal root ganglion cells in childhood at the time of chicken-pox infection, and remains there in some sort of dormant condition. Later in life, as a result of some impairment in immunological surveillance (e.g. age, immuno-suppressive treatment, lymphoma, leukaemia), the virus becomes activated and causes the features of shingles.

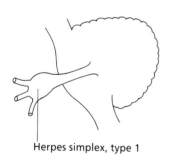

Herpes simplex, type 1

Herpes simplex infections

'Cold sores' around the mouth and nose are the commonest clinical expressions of Herpes simplex virus, *type 1* infection. A similar dormant state to that in Herpes zoster infections occurs here, with the Herpes simplex virus resident in the trigeminal nerve ganglion. The altered immunological status that accompanies another viral infection (usually a 'cold') allows the Herpes simplex virus to become activated in the ganglion, and cause the skin rash in maxillary or mandibular branch territory.

In the case of Herpes simplex virus, *type 2* infections, the site of latent infection is the dorsal root ganglion in the sacral region, and reactivation leads to *genital herpes*, in which the vesicular ulcerative lesions occur in the urogenital tract and perineal region.

Fig. 16.1. Common localized viral infections.

223   *Infections of the nervous system*

Pyogenic bacterial infections

Cerebral abscess and *spinal extradural abscess* are the consequences of localized pyogenic bacterial infection. Cerebral abscess is the more common of the two. Figure 16.2 shows the common clinical features of these two conditions.

Cerebral abscess

In the case of cerebral abscess, the continuing mortality from this condition is due to delay in diagnosis. The presence of a cerebral abscess must be anticipated whenever some of the features depicted in the upper part of Fig. 16.2 occur. In particular, the presence of one of the local infective conditions which can give rise of cerebral abscess must put one 'on guard'.

The non-specific features of an infection, i.e. fever, elevated WCC and ESR, may not be very marked in patients with cerebral abscess. Epilepsy, often with focal features, is common in patients with a brain abscess. The diagnosis should be established before the focal neurological deficit (the nature of which will depend upon the site of the abscess) and evidence of raised intracranial pressure are too severe.

Urgent CT brain scan and referral to the local neurosurgical centre are the correct lines of management of patients with suspected cerebral abscess. Lumbar puncture is contraindicated and potentially dangerous. Evacuation of pus through a burrhole, bacteriological diagnosis, and intensive antibiotic treatment are required for a successful outcome.

Spinal extradural abscess

Patients with a spinal extradural abscess present like any patient with a localized spinal cord lesion, except that pain and tenderness in the spine are often very conspicuous. The clinical picture is one that worsens very quickly. There may be clinical evidence of infection, and possibly some predisposition to infection.

Good spinal X-rays may show localized bone erosion at the site of infection. Myelography leading to decompressive surgery, organism identification (usually *Staphylococcus aureus*), and antibiotic therapy constitute the correct management.

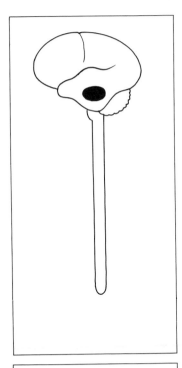

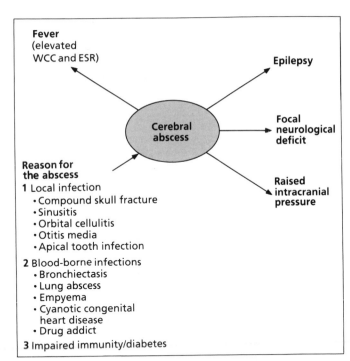

Fever
(elevated
WCC and ESR)

Epilepsy

Cerebral abscess

Focal
neurological
deficit

Raised
intracranial
pressure

Reason for the abscess
1 Local infection
 • Compound skull fracture
 • Sinusitis
 • Orbital cellulitis
 • Otitis media
 • Apical tooth infection

2 Blood-borne infections
 • Bronchiectasis
 • Lung abscess
 • Empyema
 • Cyanotic congenital
   heart disease
 • Drug addict

3 Impaired immunity/diabetes

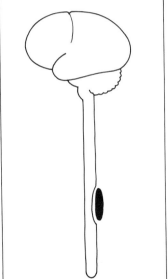

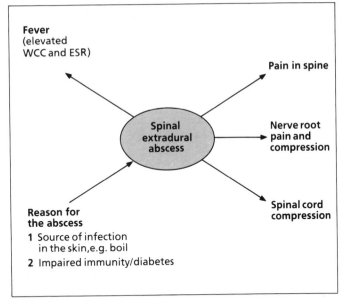

Fever
(elevated
WCC and ESR)

Pain in spine

Spinal extradural abscess

Nerve root
pain and
compression

Spinal cord
compression

Reason for the abscess
1 Source of infection
  in the skin, e.g. boil
2 Impaired immunity/diabetes

Fig. 16.2. Common localized
pyogenic bacterial infections.

Other localized infections

None of these is common in the UK.

Localized *tuberculous* infection may occur in the brain,
known as a tuberculoma. Such infections present as subacute or chronic space-occupying lesions, i.e. with epilepsy,
increasing focal neurological deficit or raised intracranial
pressure. In the spine, tuberculosis primarily infects an

intervertebral disc, then involves the adjacent vertebrae causing pain and tenderness in the spine. Unchecked, it progresses to cause nerve root pain and compression, and spinal cord compression. Tuberculous disease of this sort is seen in the immigrant population in the UK, in patients from India, Pakistan, and the West Indies.

Localized *toxoplasma* or *fungal abscesses* may occur in immuno-deficient or immuno-suppressed patients. These opportunistic infections are dealt with later in this chapter.

Common acute generalized CNS infections

Acute meningo-encephalitis is probably the best term to describe acute generalized viral or bacterial infections of the nervous system. Clinically and pathologically, there is almost always some degree of encephalitis in *acute meningitis*, and some degree of meningitis in *acute encephalitis*. Frequently, both aspects are apparent clinically. The close apposition of the meninges to the highly convoluted surface of the brain makes it very unlikely that meninges and brain

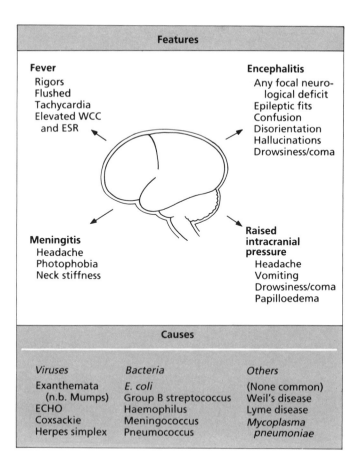

Fig. 16.3. Common acute generalized CNS infections.

tissue could escape sharing the same acute inflammatory illness.

Figure 16.3 shows the features of acute meningo-encephalitis. The emphasis on meningitic and encephalitic features varies from one patient to another, and according to the particular infecting agent. The drowsiness and coma that may occur in encephalitis may be due to associated raised intracranial pressure (brain swelling), but may alternatively indicate that the midbrain and brainstem are directly involved in the encephalitic process. The elevation of intracranial pressure may be due to brain swelling in meningo-encephalitis. Where the meningitic element is pronounced, however, CSF drainage from the ventricles back to the sagittal sinus (via the tentorial hiatus and over the surface of the brain) may become obstructed, with the development of hydrocephalus.

Viral infections

In the case of acute viral infections, the clinical picture may be of acute meningitis, acute meningo-encephalitis or acute encephalitis. A mild degree of acute meningo-encephalitis probably occurs in many acute viral infections, certainly in the common exanthematous infections of childhood, especially mumps. In adults with the clinical picture of acute viral meningo-encephalitis, the particular virus may not be identified, though ECHO and Coxsackie viruses are those most frequently responsible.

Herpes simplex encephalitis, caused by herpes virus type 1, is the most potentially lethal acute viral infection of the CNS. It can occur at any age, and produces a largely encephalitic clinical picture with or without features of raised intracranial pressure. Brain swelling, especially in the temporal regions, is common, and reflects a highly damaging and necrotic process occurring in the brain tissue. Death, or survival with a significant neurological deficit (intellectual, physical and/or epileptic), is a common sequel to this infection. Fortunately, the outcome is significantly improved if the anti-viral agent, acyclovir, is given early in the course of the disease. Unfortunately, there is no easy way of knowing, early in the course of the illness, which cases of acute encephalitis are due to Herpes simplex virus and which are due to other viruses. For this reason, any patient with acute encephalitis should receive acyclovir, especially where the infection is fulminant and producing brain swelling on CT scan. There is no evidence that acyclovir produces benefit or harm when used in patients suffering from other viral infections of the brain.

227   *Infections of the nervous system*

Bacterial infections

Acute bacterial infections of the CNS generally give rise to the clinical picture of acute meningitis (also known as bacterial meningitis, purulent meningitis and septic meningitis). It is helpful to remember, however, that these infections are meningo-encephalitic, since confusion or some alteration of the mental state, epilepsy, and drowsiness are common features of bacterial meningitis. Furthermore, it is the brain involvement that is so worrying in fulminating infections, e.g. meningococcal meningitis, which may progress to coma within hours. Persistent purulent meningitis is very likely to give rise to CSF absorption problems, so that the clinical features of raised intracranial pressure appear, along with CT scan confirmation of hydrocephalus.

In neonates, the common organisms tend to be *Escherichia coli* and Group B streptococci, but thereafter the common bacteria are *Haemophilus influenzae*, meningococcus and pneumococcus.

In all cases of bacterial meningitis, perhaps more so in adults, and especially in any case of recurrent infection, a reason for the infection must be sought. The predisposition to infection may be local, e.g.:
• head trauma involving the floor of the anterior cranial fossa, possibly with CSF rhinorrhoea;
• head trauma involving the temporal bone, with access of bacteria to the CSF from the ear;
• shunt devices *in situ* for relief of hydrocephalus;
or more general, e.g.:
• diabetes mellitus;
• immuno-deficiency or immuno-suppression.

Other infective agents

Apart from viruses and bacteria, other infective agents causing acute meningo-encephalitis are not common in the UK. Two treponemal infections, leptospirosis and Lyme disease, are occasional causes of meningitis. Meningitis may occur at the height of Weil's disease (infection with *Leptospira icterohaemorrhagica*), and the meningitis of Lyme disease is often associated with facial nerve palsy. An infection with *Myocoplasma pneumoniae* in the lungs may be complicated by a meningo-encephalitis, which is usually not too severe.

Subacute and chronic generalized CNS infections

None of these infections is common in the UK currently. This is because of comprehensive immunization of the population (tetanus, tuberculosis), of widespread frequent use of antibiotics (syphilis), or because the condition, though common elsewhere in the world, has not yet reached the UK in significant numbers (rabies, AIDS). None of the infections will be described in great detail therefore, though some awareness of each of them is certainly justified. They are listed in Fig. 16.4.

Viruses	Rabies	
	AIDS	
	Jakob-Creutzfeldt disease	
	Kuru	
	Subacute sclerosing panencephalitis	
	Progressing rubella panencephalitis	
	Progressive multifocal leucoencephalopathy	
Bacteria	Tuberculous meningitis	
	Tetanus	
	Leprosy	
Treponema	Syphilis	
Fungi	Cryptococcus	(Opportunist infections
	Candida	in patients with
	Aspergillus	impaired immunity)
Non-infective	Malignant meningitis	

Fig. 16.4. Subacute and chronic generalized CNS infections.

Rabies

This viral illness is usually contracted because the patient is bitten by an infected dog, which has the virus in its saliva. After a variable incubation period (usually 2–8 weeks, but sometimes much longer), a progressive encephalomyelitis occurs (hallucinations, apprehension, hydrophobia, flaccid paralysis with sensory and sphincter involvement), leading to bulbar and respiratory paralysis. Treatment is difficult, not very specific, prolonged and often unsuccessful.

AIDS

Apart from the predisposition to infections and certain tumours because of the immuno-deficiency resulting from the AIDS virus, there is now good evidence that the virus itself infects the CNS. This subacute encephalitis is almost certainly responsible for the 'AIDS encephalopathy', also known as the 'AIDS dementia complex'. The features of this are a slowly progressive dementia, motor and sensory dysphasia, and impairment of rapid and skilled motor activities. Pathologically, an infiltration of both grey and white matter with giant multinucleated cells of macrophage origin is found, together with foamy macrophages and reactive astrocytosis.

The AIDS virus may also directly infect the spinal cord or the peripheral nerves, to produce the clinical picture of paraplegia or peripheral neuropathy.

The most common opportunistic infections of the CNS in AIDS patients are:
- toxoplasma cerebral abscesses;
- cytomegalovirus encephalitis and retinitis;
- cryptococcal meningitis.

Jakob–Creutzfeldt disease

This progressive encephalopathy is characterized by dementia, myoclonus, cortical blindness, and paralysis, causing death within a few months in most cases. The infective agent is smaller than a virus, but has been shown to exist by transmission of the same disease to primates, using tissue from patients with the clinical disease.

It is not usually clear how an individual patient has become infected, but care with tissues from individuals with Jakob–Creutzfeldt disease is important, and with neurosurgical intruments used in their management (e.g. cerebral biopsy).

Kuru

This is a progressive and fatal cerebellar ataxia which used to occur in New Guinea. Like Jakob–Creutzfeldt disease, the illness is caused by a sub-viral transmissible agent. Unlike Jakob–Creutzfeldt disease, the source of infection in patients with kuru was obvious since cannibalism (with consumption of the brain) used to occur amongst the primitive people of New Guinea.

Subacute sclerosing panencephalitis and progressive rubella panencephalitis

After a latency of some years following measles in early childhood or congenital rubella, a slowly progressive, fatal syndrome characterized by personality change, dementia, myoclonic seizures, and ataxia occasionally occurs.

Specific anti-measles or anti-rubella antibodies become increasingly evident in the CSF during the illness, indicating the presence of viral antigen within the CNS. Brain biopsy shows eosinophilic inclusion bodies within oligodendrocytes, and electron microscopy reveals virus particles within neurones.

Progressive multifocal leuco-encephalopathy

This is a rare condition causing an accumulating number of multifocal neurological deficits, epilepsy, and dementia. It is caused by an opportunistic infection by papovavirus in patients who are immuno-deficient or immuno-suppressed.

Multiple areas of demyelination are to be found in the brain at post-mortem, with papovavirus particles in oligo-dendrocytes.

Tuberculous meningitis

This subacute form of bacterial meningitis is no longer common in the UK, but it still occurs, especially in the immigrant population. The same group of four symptoms (shown in Fig. 16.3) of acute meningo-encephalitis occur, but evolve more slowly. The meningitic process is often most evident around the base of the brain, causing cranial nerve palsies, and interfering with the return of CSF from the ventricles to the sagittal sinus. Elevated intracranial pressure and hydrocephalus are common in tuberculous meningitis.

Tetanus

This is rare in the UK because of the active and widespread immunization programme. The illness is not really an infection of the CNS, but the consequence of the neuro-toxin produced by the anaerobic bacillus, *Clostridium tetani*. This organism replicates best in a deep necrotic wound, often containing foreign material (splinters, thorn, gravel, soil). Travelling from the wound via the peripheral nerves and blood, the neurotoxin arrives in the spinal cord and brainstem, where it effectively removes inhibitory influences on the alpha motor neurones. Hypertonicity and spontaneous muscular spasms occur in the head and neck muscles (lock-jaw and the classical risus sardonicus), trunk muscles, and then the limb muscles (opisthotonus). The spasms are strong enough to cause crush fractures of the vertebrae, and prolonged enough to cause death from respiratory failure and exhaustion.

Wound excision, penicillin, tetanus antitoxin, sedation, neuromuscular blocking agents, tracheotomy and ventilation may all feature in the management of patients with tetanus.

Leprosy

In lepromatous leprosy, *Mycobacterium leprae* is present in the peripheral nerves causing a slowly progressive mononeuritis multiplex (Chapter 14, see page 183). Trophic changes in anaesthetic areas, together with muscle weakness and wasting, account for the tragic appearance of those who have had this form of leprosy for any length of time.

The condition is treatable with dapsone and certain other anti-mycobacterial drugs.

Syphilis

The central nervous system is involved in the tertiary phase of infection by the spirochaete, *Treponema pallidum*. The manifestations of neurosyphilis, which used to be common but are now very rare, are:
- optic atrophy;
- Argyll–Robertson pupils, which are small, unequal, irregular, react to accommodation but do not react to light;
- general paralysis of the insane, in which meningo-encephalitic involvement of the cerebral cortex (especially the frontal lobes, including the motor cortex) occurs. It gives rise to a combination of dementia and upper motor neurone paralysis of the limbs;
- tabes dorsalis, in which the proximal axons of the dorsal root ganglion cells, destined to travel in the posterior columns of the spinal cord, become atrophied. The clinical picture is one of proprioceptive sensory loss, especially in the legs. An unsteady, wide-based, stamping gait, and a tendency to fall in the dark, typify patients with tabes dorsalis;
- meningovascular syphilis is perhaps the most frequent clinical expression of neurosyphilis these days. The small arteries perforating the surface of the brain become inflamed and obliterated in the subacute syphilitic meningitis. Acute hemiplegia and sudden individual cranial nerve palsies are the most common clinical events in this form of the disease.

Fungi

In the main, fungal infection of the CNS is opportunistic in patients with deficient immunity. The CNS infection may occur in isolation, or in association with fungal infection of other organs, particularly the lungs. *Aspergillus, Candida* and *Cryptococcus* are the most common fungi to behave in this way, producing either chronic meningitis, or multiple cerebral abscesses, or both.

Malignant meningitis

A relentlessly progressive meningitis, often with cranial nerve and spinal nerve root lesions, and often associated with headache, pain in the spine, or root pain, may be due to infiltration of the meninges by neoplastic cells rather than infection. The neoplastic cells may be leukaemic or lymphomatous, or may be derived from a solid tumour elsewhere. Such patients are often immuno-suppressed, so the differentiation of malignant meningitis from an opportunistic infection of the meninges may be difficult. Cytological examination of the CSF may be very helpful, the malignant cells showing themselves in centrifuged CSF samples.

CNS infections in immuno-compromised patients

The prolonged survival of patients with impaired immunity is becoming more and more commonplace. The number of patients on cytotoxic drugs and steroids for the treatment of malignant disease, and to suppress immunity in connective tissue disorders and after organ transplantation, is increasing. The incidence and prevalence of AIDS are increasing.

Infections due to normal pathogens, but of increased incidence and severity	Opportunistic infections
Viruses Herpes simplex • Encephalitis Herpes zoster • Shingles • Myelitis • Encephalomyelitis	Cytomegalovirus • Encephalitis • Retinitis Papova virus • Progressive multifocal leucoencephalopathy
Bacteria Common pathogens & less common ones, e.g. pseudomonas, tuberculosis • Meningitis • Cerebral abscess	*Listeria monocytogenes* • Meningo-encephalitis
Fungi	Cryptococcus • Meningitis Candida • Meningitis • Cerebral abscesses Aspergillus • Cerebral abscesses
Protozoa	Toxoplasma • Cerebral abscess(es)

Fig. 16.5. Infections in immuno-compromised patients.

These immuno-suppressed or immuno-deficient patients are susceptible to infections:
• by organisms which are capable of causing infection in normal individuals, but which cause abnormally frequent and severe infections in the immuno-compromised;
• by organisms which are not pathogenic in normal circumstances, so called opportunistic infections.
Figure 16.5 summarizes the common CNS infections of each type.

The clinical features of these infections are often ill defined and not distinct from the patient's underlying disease. The different organisms do not create diagnostic clinical syndromes. Intensive investigation, in close collaboration with the microbiology laboratory, is usually required to establish the diagnosis and the correct treatment.

Management of infections of the nervous system

Prevent
Diagnose
Treat
Ask why

Prophylaxis

It is not trite to emphasize the importance of the preventive measures which are current in the UK to control CNS infections. We must not become lulled into complacency or lack vigilance over such matters.
• Comprehensive immunization of the population in the case of polio, tetanus, and tuberculosis.
• Measures to prevent the spread of rabies and AIDS.
• Proper care of patients with compound skull fractures, CSF rhinorrhoea and otorrhoea, otitis media, frontal sinusitis, and orbital cellulitis.
• Early active treatment of any infection in diabetic or immuno-compromised patients.

Diagnosis

Some infections will be identified from their clinical features alone, e.g. Herpes zoster.

In the case of acute meningo-encephalitis, the ideal way to establish the diagnosis is urgent CT scan (to exclude a cerebral abscess mass lesion), followed by immediate lumbar puncture. Blood count, blood culture, chest X-rays and other investigations may be helpful, but it is the CSF which is most helpful in diagnosis, as shown in Fig. 16.6.

In patients with a suspected cerebral abscess, urgent CT brain scan is the investigation of choice. Radionucleotide scanning also localizes abscesses well. If a mass lesion with the features of an abscess is found, bacteriological diagnosis is established by a needle introduced into the abscess via a

	Polymorph count ↓	Lymphocyte count ↓	Protein conc. ↓	Glucose conc. ↓	Microscopy and culture	Viral antibodies in blood and CSF
Pyogenic bacterial meningitis	↑↑↑	↑	↑	↓	+	—
Viral meningitis or meningo-encephalitis	N or ↑	↑↑	↑	N	—	+
Tuberculous meningitis	N or ↑	↑↑	↑	↓	+	—
Fungal meningitis	N or ↑	↑↑	↑	N or ↓	+	—
Cerebral abscess	Lumbar puncture should not be performed, it is potentially dangerous					

Fig. 16.6. CSF abnormalities in various CNS infections.

burrhole. Other investigations (e.g. ENT or pulmonary) to evaluate the source of infection are frequently necessary.

Treatment

Appropriate oral and intravenous antibiotic administration, usually in consultation with the microbiology laboratory, constitutes the main line of treatment for pyogenic bacterial, tuberculous, fungal, and protozoal infections.

Topical and intravenous adminstration of antiviral agents are used in Herpes simplex and zoster infections. New agents with some activity against other viruses, e.g. cytomegalovirus and AIDS, are becoming available.

General supportive measures for patients whose conscious level is depressed are often required of medical, nursing, and physiotherapy staff (Chapter 1, Fig. 1.7, see page 13).

The reason for the infection

In every patient with a CNS infection, the question must be asked 'Why has this infection occurred in this patient?'. Such a question will detect imperfections of immunization, the presence of diabetes, a state of impaired immunity, a previously undetected site of access or source for infection, a personal contact accounting for the infection, or a visit to a part of the world where the infection is endemic. Such an enquiry is an essential part of the patient's management.

235 *Infections of the nervous system*

Post-infective neurological syndromes

Figure 16.7 shows this group of conditions which involve the central or peripheral nervous system at a short interval after an infection. Guillain–Barré syndrome is probably the most common, and is fully discussed in Chapter 14.

Nature of prior infection	Target structure in the nervous system	Syndrome
Many and varied	Myelin around blood vessels in the central nervous system	Acute disseminated encephalomyelitis
Many and varied	Myelin in nerve roots, cranial nerves and peripheral nerves	Guillain-Barré syndrome
Influenza, varicella and other viruses	Mitochondria in brain and liver	Reye's syndrome
Coxsackie B, and other viruses	?? What's wrong	Myalgic encephalomyelitis
Group A streptococcus	Basal ganglia	Sydenham's chorea

Fig. 16.7. Post-infective neurological syndromes.

Acute disseminated encephalomyelitis

Days or weeks after an infection or immunization, a multifocal perivascular allergic reaction in the CNS, associated with perivascular demyelination, may occur.

The clinical expression of such an occurrence varies from mild features of an acute encephalomyelitis, to more major focal or multifocal neurological deficits, to a life-threatening or fatal syndrome with epileptic seizures, major bilateral neurological signs, ataxia, brainstem signs, and coma.

Acute cerebellar ataxia of young children may have the same underlying pathological mechanism.

Guillain–Barré syndrome

In this condition (fully described in Chapter 14, see page 196), the post-infectious immunological lesion affects the spinal nerve roots, and the cranial and peripheral nerves.

There is damage to the myelin which is under the care of Schwann cells. After a phase of damage, which may show itself by progressive weakness and numbness over 1–4 weeks, the clinical state and pathological process stabilize, with subsequent gradual recovery.

Recovery from Guillain–Barré syndrome is usually complete, whereas persistent deficits are not uncommon after severe acute disseminated encephalomyelitis. Schwann cells can reconstitute peripheral nerve and nerve root myelin with much greater efficiency than oligodendrocytes can repair myelin within the central nervous system.

Reye's syndrome

In this condition, which occurs in young children, there is damage to the brain and liver in the wake of a viral infection, (especially influenza and varicella). Treatment of the child's infection with aspirin seems to raise the chances of developing Reye's syndrome (so avoidance of the use of aspirin in young children has been recommended).

Vomiting is a common early persistent symptom, rapidly progressing to coma, seizures, bilateral neurological signs, and evidence of raised intracranial pressure due to cerebral oedema.

The primary insult seems to involve mitochondrial function in both brain and liver. Abnormal liver function is evident on investigation, with hypoglycaemia, which may clearly aggravate the brain lesion.

Myalgic encephalomyelitis

A very small number of patients enters into a most miserable and protracted clinical state following a viral infection. Extreme tiredness, and reduced exercise tolerance, with muscle aches and pains develop. The condition may last for months, but more usually years.

The status of this illness is not yet fully established. It may not, of course, be a single entity. In some instances, it may be entirely or predominantly psychosomatic. On the other hand, it may reflect an impaired immunological response to a viral infection with persistent viral residence in the body. Amongst the support for the viral infection theory, available evidence seems to implicate Coxsackie B infection.

Sydenham's chorea (St Vitus' dance)

When group A streptococcal sore throats were common in children, chorea (often associated with some alteration in the mental and emotional state) used to be seen 1–4 weeks later. The syndrome used to last for a few weeks, and then settle, with occasional relapses.

Rheumatic fever and a raised anti-streptolysin O titre in the blood were frequent accompaniments.

The condition is very rare now. The precise pathogenesis remains unknown.

Chapter 17　　　Psychological aspects of neurology

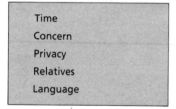

Time

Concern

Privacy

Relatives

Language

Communication

One of the main functions of a neurologist is to allow the occurrence of a neurological illness in a patient to be managed as straightforwardly as possible. This means the establishment of the correct diagnosis without undue delay, proper management of the illness, and good explanation of the diagnosis and management to the patient, to the family, and to the other doctors and health professionals who are involved in the case.

The patient and family should be able to share in the formulation of the management plan, and plenty of opportunity should be given for them to express their feelings about the symptoms, diagnosis, neurological deficit, investigations, and treatment.

Throughout the doctor's contact with an individual patient's illness, the following five points are helpful from the communication point of view. The doctor should show, in an open and friendly way, that:

1 there is always enough time;

2 there is always enough concern;

3 enough privacy is always available for the patient to speak freely and openly;

4 there is always an opportunity to talk to the patient's family;

5 he can talk to the patient and family in language they can easily understand.

Such behaviour in the doctor is required not only during information collection, i.e. in the establishment of the diagnosis, and in the assessment of the patient's reaction to his illness. It is equally necessary when the time comes to explain the nature of the illness, the treatment required, and the consequences of both for the patient.

Investment of such time and effort on a patient with a neurological illness is always worthwhile. The more the patient and family trust, like, and respect the doctor, the greater will be their confidence in the diagnosis and their compliance with the management. For example:

- 'You're OK, there doesn't seem to be anything for you to worry about, the symptoms don't have any serious cause.'
- 'It is Parkinson's disease but we can almost certainly help you quite a bit, though it will probably mean taking pills every day.'

It is clearly a shame when a doctor is knowledgeable and intelligent, but lacks the communication skills to be completely acceptable to patients under his care. Figure 17.1 is a simplified illustration of the importance of both knowledge and communication skills.

Finally, it is important to remember communication between doctors, e.g. hospital staff and family doctors, and between doctors and other health professionals (nurses, physiotherapists, etc.). It is worthwhile taking the trouble to make sure that all those involved in the management of a patient know the diagnosis and treatment plan. This helps to keep everybody interested in the case, and prevents the patient becoming confused by contradictory information.

	Good communication skills	Bad communication skills
Clever and well-informed	A good doctor	A shame, because patients will not take enough notice of this doctor
Unintelligent and ill-informed	A dangerous doctor, patients will follow his bad advice	A completely ineffective doctor, he knows nothing but nobody pays any attention to what he says

Fig. 17.1. The importance of knowledge and communication skills in a doctor.

An abnormal psychological reaction may originate from:
- the patient's personality
- the patient's perception of the illness as something too great for him to master

Psychological reactions to neurological illness

In this section, we are recognizing that the total illness in any patient is the sum of the physical illness plus the patient's psychological reaction to the physical illness. The latter may be appropriate and entirely understandable. Sometimes, however, the reaction is exaggerated for some reason, making the whole illness a bigger one for the patient, his family, and for the medical staff looking after him. Recognition of the two elements of illness, and the management of both, are particularly appropriate in patients with neurological disorders. This is because some of the illnesses generate a good deal of concern in most people, e.g. grand mal epileptic attacks, and also because some neurological illnesses are physically disabling but lack specific

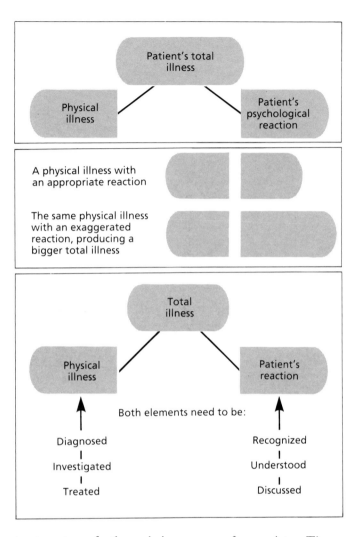

Fig. 17.2. The importance of a patient's psychological reaction to a physical illness.

treatment, a further obvious cause for anxiety. These elements of illness and management are illustrated in Fig. 17.2.

There are two broad reasons for an abnormal psychological reaction.

1 In general, patients tend to tackle physical illness with the same *personality* characteristics that they use to tackle any other of life's challenges. The patient invokes the coping processes that he usually employs to deal with stress. In most instances, the patient copes well, but sometimes the personality allows too massive a reaction, so that the patient:
- becomes over-dependent;
- tries to control the illness and management very rigidly himself;
- dramatizes and becomes too emotionally moved by the illness;

- adopts an unnecessarily long-suffering or self-sacrificial response;
- becomes too resentful;
- tries to deny the presence of the illness;
- becomes pre-occupied with the illness;
- becomes anxious;
- becomes depressed.

2 Anxiety, depression, prolongation of the sick role, and other psychological reactions may occur in the patient, not because of his pre-existing personality, but because *the physical illness is perceived by him as something too great for him to master.* For him, the illness or its consequences may appear to be:

- *too great a loss:*
'I can't even walk straight, and have to hold onto the bannisters on stairs like an old man.'
'Work's going to be hard with hands like these, and I certainly don't see how I can keep up my fishing.'
'I don't see how I can get through two whole years without driving.'

- *too great a threat:*
'My uncle had headaches like these, and dropped down dead with a brain haemorrhage when he was 40.'
'My marriage is a little shaky anyway, I shouldn't think he'll stay with me now he knows I've got MS.'
'I never thought a chap like me would come to depend on pills every day for the rest of his life.'

- *too great a gain:*
'The accident wasn't my fault. Now I have headaches, epilepsy, and some weakness of my left arm. I can't work and need compensation.'
'Now that I have peripheral neuropathy as well as diabetes and blood pressure, he's going to have to stop going out so much and look after me.'

An experienced neurologist is assessing the patient's psychological reaction to his symptoms, and to the investigations, diagnosis, and suggested management, throughout his contact with the patient. The feelings and reactions occurring in the patient's family are also very important, since they can strongly modify what goes on in the patient's mind. Giving time for listening, understanding, discussion, explanation, and support is the key to helping patients in their reaction to a neurological illness. It is often possible to improve an abnormal reaction in this way.

Neurological presentations of psychological illness

There should be two features of the patient's illness to suggest that there is little or no physical disease present, and that the symptoms are symptomatic of a psychological disorder.

1 The patient's description of his symptoms should not sound like those of a physical illness, and may positively suggest a non-organic syndrome (e.g. 'a tight band sensation around my head, present all the time, and unrelieved by any painkillers' — tension headache). Physical examination should be negative.

2 There should be some evidence of the underlying psychological disorder. The assessment of the patient's personality, and the detection of the common psychological conditions, *anxiety* and *depression*, are functions of the initial interview with the patient.

The following are common neurological presentations of psychological diseases.

Anxiety

- Tension headache (Chapter 3, see page 36).
- Muscular tension causing neck pain, shoulder pain, back pain.
- Tremor (Chapter 9, see page 107).
- Hyperventilation causing dizziness, blackouts, and mouth and limb sensory symptoms (Chapter 1, see page 4).
- Irreconcilable concern, becoming an obsession or phobia, about one symptom, e.g. tinnitus having a serious treatable cause, or about one specific disease being present, e.g. syphilis, multiple sclerosis, myasthenia or AIDS.
- Heightened focus upon a normal physiological phenomenon, e.g. tremor in the hands or fasciculation in the calves after exercise.

Depression

- Pseudo-dementia (Chapter 4, see page 46).
- Pains in the face (Chapter 3, see page 43), and elsewhere in the body. It is probable that pain thresholds can be altered by mood, in terms of altered neuro-transmission in the root entry zone in the dorsal columns of the spinal cord.
- Physical retardation, exhaustion, lack of normal energy and enthusiasm may be the paramount features in some cases of depression.

Hysteria and malingering

- Episodes of amnesia.
- Episodes of loss of consciousness.
- Inability to speak.
- Inability to see.
- Loss of use and feeling in:
  an arm;
  a leg;
  an arm and a leg;
  both legs.

How useful the words hysteria and malingering are remains questionable. They usually give rise to offence in patients who find that such diagnoses have been put in their case notes. Hysteria suggests subconscious production of physical disability without any physical cause. Malingering suggests conscious production of physical disability without any physical cause. In practice, it is usually very difficult to know whether the process is a subconscious or conscious one, and not infrequently there is an underlying minor physical abnormality which is exaggerated by the patient.

Certainly, the two factors that give rise to an exaggerated reaction to physical illness (personality, or sense of loss, threat or gain, referred to in the previous section of this chapter) are highly relevant when one is dealing with patients with a disability in which the underlying physical abnormality is small or non-existent.

The clues that there may be a major functional, i.e. non-physical, element in a patient's neurological syndrome are:

- evidence of personality disorder, or obvious reason why the patient might perceive the disability as an extraordinary loss, threat, or gain. This may be much more subtle than a straightforward post-accident compensation situation;
- evidence of multiple previous functional illnesses, where no underlying physical cause for symptoms has been found;
- marked variability or inconsistency in the neurological disability, e.g. palpable variability in power during the neurological examination, or a much worse disability during medical rounds and examinations than when the patient is getting about the ward 'unobserved' for eating, dressing, and toilet purposes. During the assessment of power in the neurological examination, there may be simultaneous contraction of antagonist muscles with the agonists — an excess of effort for little accomplished movement;
- great sensitivity in the patient and family that the problem is psychologically, rather than physically, mediated.

243 *Psychological aspects of neurology*

Management of such cases is not easy and requires:
- a great deal of time, self-control and effort on the part of the doctor;
- that the doctor, patient, and family reach a state of confidence that there is no major continuing physical disease present;
- a search to understand why the patient has reacted in this way. Is the exaggerated functional disability comprehensible in terms of the patient's personality? Are there continuing reasons why the patient should find the sick role rewarding? There is not much a doctor can do to change the patient's personality, but discussion may help to change the patient's perception of his disability in terms of loss, threat, or gain;
- a genuine wish on the part of the patient to recover from the disability;
- fairly lengthy and intensive physical rehabilitation by the doctor and physiotherapists;
- counselling of the patient to help him to avoid 'losing face' for having such an illness, to set his sights on nothing less than 100% recovery, and to re-adjust the attitudes of the family to accept the patient as a healthy robust person again rather than an invalid requiring special care and attention.

Conditions in the borderland between neurology and psychiatry

Acute confusional state

Post-concussion syndrome

Post-viral syndrome i.e. Myalgic encephalomyelitis

Alcohol and drug related disorders

Dementia

An *acute confusional state*, with disorientation, hallucinations, incomprehensible speech, and restlessness, always gives rise to concern. Such a patient may be admitted to psychiatric hospital because the family doctor and psychiatrist feel that the patient has an acute psychiatric disorder. This may be quite correct. The common physical disorders which can give rise to this acute clinical picture are:
- a febrile illness, especially in the young and old;
- drugs, especially in the elderly;
- dysphasia, especially a fluent sensory dysphasia (Chapter 15, see page 208), due to a lesion in the dominant temporal lobe;
- repeated temporal lobe epileptic attacks (Chapter 2, see page 23);
- meningo-encephalitis, especially viral encephalitis (Chapter 16, see page 226).

In both the *post-concussion syndrome* (Chapter 8, see page 102), and the *post-viral syndrome* (Chapter 16, see page 237), there is a combination of neurological and psychiatric symptoms. Depression and impaired cerebral or neuro-muscular function are the characteristic features of these fairly stereotyped clinical syndromes. The underlying pathological process is conjectural in both.

Alcohol-induced damage to the CNS (Chapter 4, see page 51) is often diagnosed by neurologists, but best managed by psychiatrists with experience in drink-related problems. The *drug-induced disorders of movement* that accompany prolonged use of the major tranquillizers (Chapter 9, see page 113) often require the intervention of the neurologist in a patient under the ongoing care of a psychiatrist.

The provision of custodial care for the increasing number of patients suffering from *dementia*, whether non-progressive in nature (e.g. after head injury), or progressive from whatever cause (Chapter 4, see page 50), is a major challenge to both neurologists and psychiatrists — a challenge that has not yet been adequately met.

Index